Royal Society of Medicine

International Congress and Symposium Series

Number 3

Stress-free Anaesthesia

Analgesia and the Suppression
of Stress Responses

*Proceedings of an International Symposium held by the Janssen
Research Foundation at Beerse, Belgium on 10 February 1978*

Royal Society of Medicine

International Congress and Symposium Series

Number 3

Stress-free Anaesthesia

Analgesia and the Suppression
of Stress Responses

Edited by
C. WOOD

1978

Published jointly by

THE ROYAL SOCIETY OF MEDICINE
1 Wimpole Street, London

ACADEMIC PRESS
London

GRUNE & STRATTON
New York

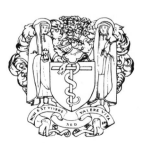

ROYAL SOCIETY OF MEDICINE
1 Wimpole Street, London W1M 8AE

ACADEMIC PRESS INC. (LONDON) LTD.
24/28 Oval Road, London NW1 7DX

United States Edition published and distributed by
GRUNE & STRATTON INC,
111 Fifth Avenue, New York, New York 10013

Library of Congress Catalog Card Number: 78-67902
ISBN (Academic Press): 0-12-763350-2
ISBN (Grune & Stratton): 0-8089-1135-X

Printed in Great Britain by Staples Printers Rochester Limited at The Stanhope Press.

Contributors

C. Conseiller
Hôpital Ambroise Paré, Boulogne-Billancourt, France

J. Crul
Department of Anaesthesiology, Catholic University of Nijmegen, Netherlands

R. Dudziak
University Clinic, Department of Anaesthesiology, Frankfurt-on-Main, West Germany

D. Duvaldestin
Anaesthesia Service, Hôpital Bichat, Paris, France

A. Florence
Broadgreen Hospital, Liverpool, UK

P. Glaser
Department of Anaesthesiology, Hôpital Pitié Salpetrière, Paris, France

G. M. Hall
Department of Anaesthetics, Hammersmith Hospital, London, UK

D. Kettler
Institute for Clinical Anaesthesiology, University of Goettingen, West Germany

E. Martin
University Institute for Anaestnesiology, Munich, West Germany

E. Mathews
The Queen Elizabeth Hospital, Birmingham, UK

O. Mayrhofer
Vienna General Hospital, Austria

E. Ott
University Institute for Anaesthesiology, Munich, West Germany

K. Peter
University Institute for Anaesthesiology, Munich, West Germany

C. Prys-Roberts
Department of Anaesthetics, Royal Infirmary, Bristol, UK

R. S. Reneman
Department of Physiology, University of Limburg, Maastricht, Netherlands

Contributors

T. Savege

Anaesthetics Unit, The London Hospital, London, UK

W. Soudijn

Department of Pharmaceutical Chemistry, University of Amsterdam, Roeterseiland, Amsterdam, Netherlands

T. H. Stanley

Department of Anesthesiology, University of Utah College of Medicine, Salt Lake City, USA

P. Viars

Department of Anaesthesiology, Hôpital Pitié Salpetrière, Paris, France

B. Walton

Anaesthetic Unit, The London Hospital, London, UK

H. J. Wüst

University Institute for Anaesthesiology, Dusseldorf, West Germany

M. Zindler

University Institute for Anaesthesiology, Dusseldorf, West Germany

Contents

Chairman's Introduction

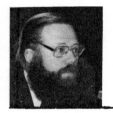

R. S. RENEMAN

*Department of Physiology, University of Limburg,
Maastricht, Netherlands*

In the past decades several techniques have been developed in anaesthesia which make use of intravenous compounds. Among these techniques, neuroleptanalgesia or NLA has become popular, mainly because of the stable situation created by this technique. More recently, however, several anaesthesiologists have changed the NLA technique to some extent by decreasing the doses of droperidol or even deleting droperidol altogether, whilst significantly increasing the dose of fentanyl, even up to $25–50\mu g/kg$ i.v.

Invariably, new techniques prompt queries and with regard to high doses of fentanyl several questions can certainly be raised. For example, why is this technique better than classical NLA and how sure are we that giving high doses of fentanyl really produces a distress-free situation? Indeed, how do we measure distress? It is also necessary to enquire about muscle relaxation and hypnosis with this technique and a last very practical question concerns post-operative assisted ventilation and hence the applicability of the technique in a general hospital setting.

These papers answer at least some of these questions, because the contributors are all experts in the field and have experience, both with classical NLA techniques and with relatively high doses of fentanyl.

*Stress-free Anaesthesia: Royal Society of Medicine International Congress and Symposium Series No. 3,
published jointly by Academic Press Inc. (London) Ltd., and the Royal Society of Medicine.*

The Pharmacology and the Pharmacokinetics of Fentanyl

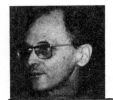

W. SOUDIJN

Department of Pharmaceutical Chemistry,
University of Amsterdam, Netherlands

With the chemical structure of morphine in mind, a very large number of chemical congeners have been synthesized and screened for analgesic properties. The route to highly potent synthetic opiates, however, was uncovered with the discovery that pethidine, originally designed as an atropine-like agent, possessed analgesic activity but with a potency of 0·5 of that of morphine in animal experiments. The chemical structure shows similarity with the structure of morphine (Fig. 1). A considerable increase in potency (2×morphine) was obtained with the reversed ester, in which

Figure 1. Chemical structure of: (a) morphine, (b, c) pethidine, (d) reversed ester of pethidine, (e) fentanyl.

Stress-free Anaesthesia: Royal Society of Medicine International Congress and Symposium Series No. 3, published jointly by Academic Press Inc. (London) Ltd., and the Royal Society of Medicine.

the C=O group and the O atom of pethidine were switched. Both compounds have a slow onset and a prolonged duration of action, because the speed of their passage through lipid membranes (which is dependent on the ratio of lipid solubility to water solubility) is comparatively small.

In fentanyl, a chemical congener of the reversed ester (Fig. 1), this ratio is shifted towards a higher value by an increase of lipid solubility. When the ratio reaches an optimal value, penetration through physiological lipid barriers is very rapid and the result is a rapid onset and a limited duration of action, when the drug is not specifically bound and retained by the target tissue. Easy penetration through lipid barriers also

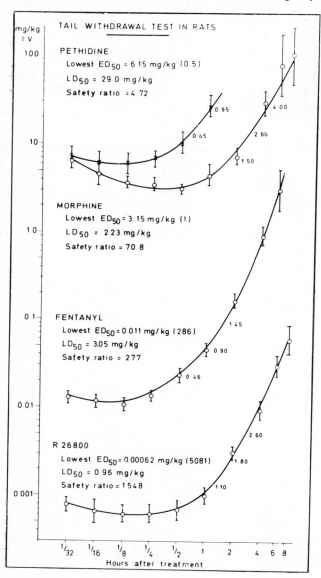

Figure 2. Tail withdrawal test in male Wistar rats ED₅₀ for effect > 10 sec after i.v. injection of pethidine, morphine, fentanyl and R26800 against time.

results in higher concentrations of the drug at the receptor sites with the consequence that the potency of the drug is increased. Fentanyl is 286 times more potent than morphine in animal experiments.

The analgesic potency of the drug is measured by the tail withdrawal reaction test in rats, as described by Janssen *et al.* (1963). When the tail of a naive rat is immersed in water at 55°C, the rat withdraws its tail within 6 sec. A drug is considered to have a moderate effect when the tail withdrawal time is more than 6 sec but less than 10 sec and a pronounced effect when there is no tail withdrawal response within 10 sec.

In Fig. 2, the ED_{50} necessary to evoke a pronounced analgesic effect after i.v. administration of pethidine, morphine, fentanyl and R26800, a very potent fentanyl derivative, is plotted against time. From the data, it is concluded that fentanyl is much more potent than morphine and pethidine and that fentanyl has a shorter duration of action, because the slope of the curve is much steeper than that of the morphine and pethidine curves. The safety ratio for fentanyl appears to be larger (277) than that of either morphine (70·8) or pethidine (4·7). When given orally, in the dosage range 0·11–1·62 mg/kg in the same test, fentanyl is about ten times less potent than when administered intravenously (Janssen *et al.*, 1963; Fig. 3).

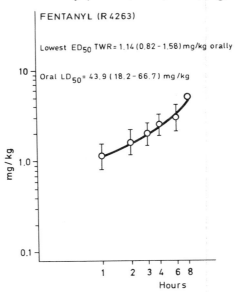

FENTANYL (R 4263)

Lowest ED_{50} TWR = 1.14 (0.82 – 1.58) mg/kg orally

Oral LD_{50} = 43.9 (18.2 – 66.7) mg/kg

Figure 3. Tail withdrawal test in male Wistar rats ED$_{50}$ for effect > 10 sec after oral administration of fentanyl against time.

To explain the unexpectedly prolonged duration of action of fentanyl in patients in comparison to rats, some authors suggest that fentanyl (by analogy with pethidine) is sequestered in the stomach during operation and is reabsorbed after passage into the small intestine. This seems unlikely to be correct since the doses used clinically are low; only a part of the administered fentanyl finds its way into the stomach; the drug, after absorption from the small intestine, has to pass through the liver where it is metabolized to a certain extent before it reaches the central nervous system and the oral potency of fentanyl is low.

In animal experiments using tritium-labelled fentanyl administered i.v. to male Wistar rats (0·31 mg/kg) it was shown that the compound was very rapidly metabolized and excreted. Most of the drug, plus its metabolites, were excreted within 24 h and the excretion appeared approximately equally distributed between the urine and the faeces (Fig. 4). About 25% of the fentanyl was excreted unchanged, mainly in the faeces.

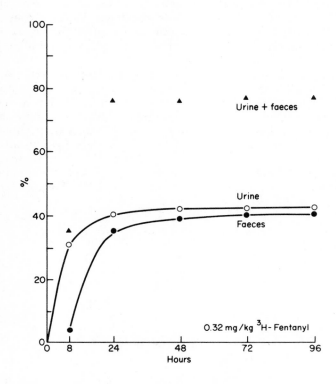

Figure 4. *Percentage of administered radioactivity excreted with the urine and faeces in male Wistar rats after i.v. injection of tritium-labelled fentanyl (0·31 mg/kg) against time.*

The major metabolic pathway appeared to be oxidative *N*-dealkylation (Fig. 5) resulting in the formation of phenylacetic acid, which is also an intermediate in the catabolism of phenylalanine and a basic metabolite, which itself is devoid of analgesic properties.

Another possible metabolic pathway was found by Maruyama and Hosoya (1969) who administered very high doses (3·5 mg/kg) of unlabelled fentanyl s.c. to female rats and detected another basic metabolite (Fig. 6) which is also pharmacologically inactive. It may well be that this product is only formed when the oxidative *N*-dealkylation pathway is saturated. There is ample experimental evidence that the liver is the main organ for the biotransformation of fentanyl.

Fentanyl is also extensively and rapidly metabolized in man, but apart from the fact that the metabolites are very water soluble, nothing is known about their chemical structure. It is well known, however, that oxidative *N*-dealkylation is a usual pathway for the biotransformation of drugs in man also.

The pharmacokinetics of tritium-labelled fentanyl were studied in the Wistar rat after i.v. injection of 0·31 mg/kg. Within 15 min a peak concentration was reached

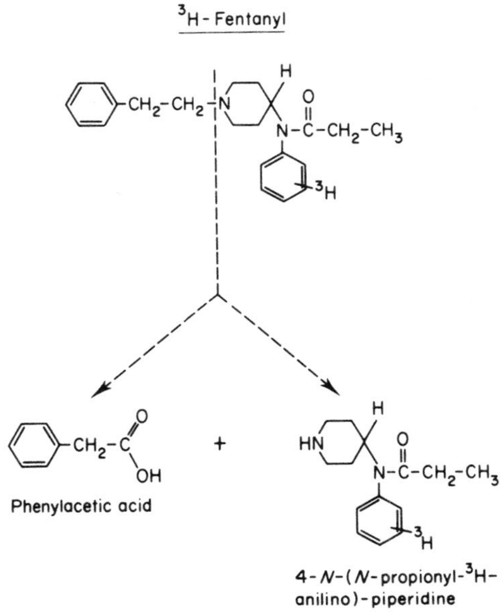

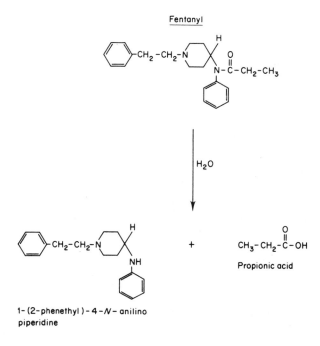

³H- Fentanyl
CH2-CH2-N
H
O
N-C-CH2-CH3
3H
CH2-C
O
OH
+
HN
H
O
N-C-CH2-CH3
3H
Phenylacetic acid
4-N-(N-propionyl-³H-anilino)-piperidine

Figure 5. Oxidative N-dealkylation of fentanyl.

Fentanyl
CH2 -CH2-N
H
O
N-C-CH2-CH3
H2O
CH2-CH2-N
H
NH
+
O
CH3-CH2-C-OH
Propionic acid
1-(2-phenethyl)-4-N-anilino piperidine

Figure 6. Alternative pathway of the biodegradation of fentanyl.

in the brain and liver. Up to 30 min after the injection, more than 95% of the radio-activity of the brain and blood was due to fentanyl itself, but 15 min after injection, substantial amounts of metabolites were already present in the liver, indicating a rapid biodegradation of the drug in rats. Half an hour after the injection, the elimination of fentanyl starts in the liver, brain and blood. The slopes of the elimination part of the curves are virtually parallel, indicating an identical half-life of fentanyl in the organs under observation (Fig. 7). There is a rapid rise in metabolite concentration

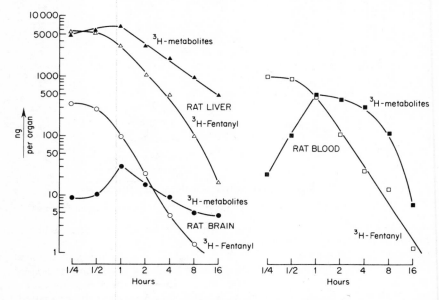

Figure 7. Pharmacokinetics of fentanyl (0·31 mg/kg, i.v.) and its radioactive metabolites in the male Wistar rat.

in the brain and in the blood in the first 60 min. Thereafter, the metabolites are eliminated from the organs at a slower rate than the elimination rate of fentanyl.

Hess et al. (1971) found that in rabbits, fentanyl is rapidly eliminated from the plasma after i.v. injection. Within 5 min, 99% of the administered dose had already disappeared from the plasma. At 0·5 min, 24% of the dose was found in the lung, while at the same time the highest brain concentration was reached, about 1% of the dose. The lung has a depot function for the redistribution of fentanyl for about 5–10 min after administration of the drug.

The paucity of publications on the pharmacokinetics of fentanyl in man is under-standable, because labelled fentanyl is required, which precludes research on a large number of subjects. However, with the development of a sensitive and specific radio-immunoassay for fentanyl (Henderson et al., 1975; Michiels et al., 1977) this situation will certainly improve and more reports will probably appear in the near future. The data published so far show a triphasic disappearance of fentanyl from serum or plasma. The initial phase is very rapid with a half-life of about 2 min. The drug is taken up by organs with a large blood supply, e.g. lung, kidney, heart and brain. The next phase is one of redistribution and the plasma half-life of fentanyl is about 10 min, the redistribution from lung, kidney and heart being more important than from the brain. The last phase is that of metabolism and excretion with a half-life of plasma fentanyl of about 172 min (Fig. 8). The above mentioned kinetics do not appear to depend on dose. Michiels and co-workers showed that in healthy volunteers the plasma level of fentanyl 2 min after an i.v. bolus injection of 0·2 mg was only

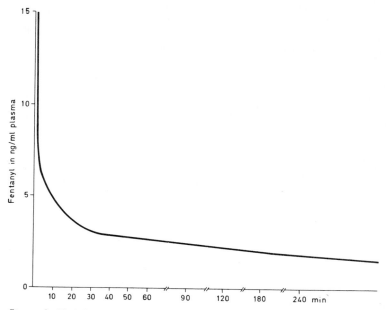

Figure 8. Model curve of the plasma fentanyl concentration against time.

2 ng/ml, 95% of the administered dose being taken up by the tissues, while 6 h after the administration, the plasma level was about 0·2 ng/ml.

Mathematically, the pharmacokinetics of fentanyl in man are best described by a three compartment open model, in which V_1 is a central (e.g. plasma+extracullular water) compartment, V_2 and V_3 are peripheral (tissue) compartments and K_{12} and K_{13} are intercompartmental rate constants. The parameters can be estimated by the method of Hull and McLeod (1976).

Bower *et al.* (1976) showed that there is a large variability in the compartmental volumes and rate constants which is not related to body mass or surface area when fentanyl was administered to eight healthy volunteers (0·2 mg i.v.).

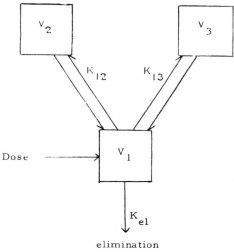

$V_1 = 59·5 \pm 46·1$; $V_2 = 71·7 \pm 61·2$; $V_3 = 189·4 \pm 97·6$ litres;
$K_{12} = 3·9 \pm 3·8$; $K_{13} = 2·12 \pm 0·9$ h^{-1}

Figure 9. Three compartment pharmacokinetic models for fentanyl.

There was also a wide variation of drug clearance between subjects. At present it is not possible to predict the duration of action of fentanyl from estimation of its plasma level in an individual patient. Even when the analysis can be performed in a very short time there will always be a delay in carrying it out.

Acknowledgement

I wish to thank Dr C. J. E. Niemegeers for providing the pharmacological data.

References

Bower, S., Holland, D. E. and Hull, C. J. (1976). *British Journal of Anaesthesia* **48,** 1121.
Henderson, G. L., Fincke, J., Leung, C. Y., Torten, M. and Benjamin, E. (1975). *Journal of Pharmacology and Experimental Therapeutics* **192,** 489.
Hess, R., Herz, A. and Friedel, K. (1971). *Journal of Pharmacology and Experimental Therapeutics* **179,** 474.
Hull, C. J. and McLeod, K. (1976). *British Journal of Anaesthesia* **48,** 677.
Janssen, P. A. J., Niemegeers, C. J. E. and Dony, J. G. H. (1963). *Arzneimittel Forschung* **13,** 502.
Maruyama, Y. and Hosoya, E. (1969) *Keio Journal of Medicine* **18,** 59.
Michiels, M., Hendriks, R. and Heykants, J. (1977). *European Journal of Clinical Pharmacology* **12,** 153

Discussion
R. S. Reneman (*Chairman*)

What is the fraction bound to plasma proteins?

W. Soudijn

The fraction is about 80–90%. The binding to proteins must be very weak because fentanyl disappears very quickly from the plasma.

Reduction or Obliteration of Reflex Responses to Surgery

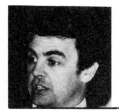

T. SAVEGE

Anaesthetics Unit, London Hospital, UK

It has long been known that anaesthesia is associated with cardiovascular changes, both pressor and depressor. When the muscle relaxant drugs were introduced and so-called light anaesthesia became fashionable, these responses became more obvious. Even in 1949 there was discussion about changes in the cardiovascular system during this technique of anaesthesia and suggestions that it was important to give small doses of pethidine to prevent changes in heart rate and blood pressure. In 1956, a review of the various techniques used to prevent cardiovascular changes and augment muscle relaxant anaesthesia suggested that one of the problems was uncertainty about how often analgesic drugs should be given and at what doses they should be administered.

The problem is still with us. In a paper in the *British Journal of Anaesthesia* in 1976, Holmes made exactly the same comment. Furthermore, we know that these cardio-vascular reflexes still occur in anaesthesia. Since the 1940s there has been a consider-able number of reports on the cardiovascular changes at intubation, resulting in increases in blood pressure, in heart rate and a relatively high incidence of dysrhyth-mias, of the order of 20%. Many who have written on this subject have claimed that patients did not come to any definite harm. On the other hand, all agree that these effects are undesirable and might have unpleasant consequences for a patient with cardiovascular disease. Bradycardias and hypotension are also known to occur during anaesthesia as a result of reflex responses and Loder, as long ago as 1947, suggested infiltrating autonomic ganglia in the abdominal cavity during the course of a laparotomy.

Like most anaesthetists we have seen cardiovascular changes during abdominal surgery. For example, a patient having a cholecystectomy, anaesthetized with althesin as an induction agent, nitrous oxide, oxygen, and intermittent small doses of fentanyl, responded to surgical stimulation by developing a marked fall in heart rate followed shortly afterwards by a fall in blood pressure. The bradycardia is presumably due to a vagal reflex response. It is interesting that once the blood pressure falls, the heart rate rises above the resting rate, suggesting that the baroreceptors sense the fall in blood pressure and override the vagal response. Blood pressure was restored spon-taneously and the anaesthetist started halothane, but some 10 min later another

Stress-free Anaesthesia: Royal Society of Medicine International Congress and Symposium Series No. 3, published jointly by Academic Press Inc. (London) Ltd., and the Royal Society of Medicine.

stimulus occurred, occasioning exactly similar changes in blood pressure and heart rate. The cerebral function monitor trace showed a dip in measured voltage co-incidental with each stimulus. Thus, when a noxious stimulus produces reflex cardiovascular changes it may have some effect on the cortex as well, even though the patient is anaesthetized.

The cardiovascular effects of a noxious stimulus during anaesthesia are well known and the purpose of administering an analgesic drug appears to be two-fold, first to reduce these noxious responses and secondly, to provide some analgesia into the post-operative phase. It is the first indication which seems most imprecise. The question is, to what extent should we attenuate these noxious responses? Should we completely obliterate them or merely limit their extent? What other widespread reactions occur at the same time; are they harmful to the patient and how are we to monitor these responses?

I believe that the intermittent measurement of blood pressure and heart rate is almost certainly unreliable because it does not reveal variations in heart rate and blood pressure effectively. It is also true that anaesthetists usually welcome a rise in blood pressure when a knife is put into the patient's abdomen. Very often the blood pressure is low after induction and the stimulus of the incision brings it back to a normal level. But this may not mean that all is well.

We are interested in this problem because we have been developing a total intravenous anaesthetic technique using an infusion of althesin, intermittent fentanyl and muscle relaxation and ventilating the patient with air and added oxygen. We noticed that although these patients were clearly unconscious as judged by the cerebral function monitor, there were often marked cardiovascular responses to noxious stimulation during the surgery.

Before describing our study in detail it is necessary to explain the use of the cerebral function monitor (Fig. 1). This instrument measures the EEG from a single pair of

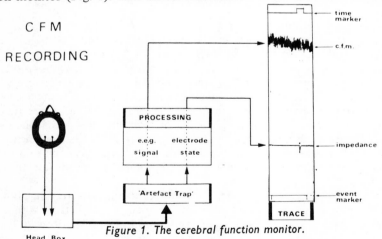

Figure 1. The cerebral function monitor.

electrodes. It is designed to produce the EEG in a compressed, relatively filtered form, which can be easily interpreted. The trace on the paper is a smoothed curve of voltage between the two electrodes. If the trace is high then it reflects high cortical energy. Conversely, if the trace is low, it reflects low cortical energy. If the trace is very wide, this suggests a very wide variation of energy.

Figure 2 is an example of the response to barbiturate drugs for example. With the patient awake the cerebral function monitor shows normal activity. Induction of

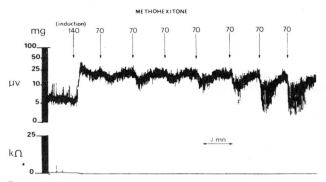

Figure 2. Cerebral function response to barbiturates.

anaesthesia produces a characteristic increase in cortical energy which is seen with all induction agents. The patient goes to sleep and the trace moves down and gets broader as the cortex becomes more depressed. One bolus dose, of course, does not last for long and as the patient starts to recover a second dose is given (half the induction dose) which depresses the trace again. Subsequent incremental doses of methohexitone are all equally spaced. Thus the cerebral function monitor can be used to see how deeply the cortex is depressed by the anaesthetic. The cortex becomes progressively more depressed and this progressive suppression seen for longer periods after each dose suggests accumulation.

We have been anaesthetizing patients with an althesin infusion to keep them unconscious, giving them a muscle relaxant and ventilating them with air, and following the cerebral function monitor to establish how deeply anaesthetized they are in terms of cortical depression. We measure arterial blood pressure and pulse rate continuously. We apply a noxious stimulus (a pressure on the skin over the tibia) while the patient is unconscious and measure the change in blood pressure and pulse rate. Subsequently variable doses of fentanyl are administered. The stimulus is repeated and the changes again measured. A small dose of methoxamine is given before and after each experiment to check that the peripheral vasculature is still able to constrict and has not in any way been affected by the dose of fentanyl.

An example of the record obtained is shown in Fig. 3. During the course of the recording the CFM trace gradually became broader and nearer to the baseline,

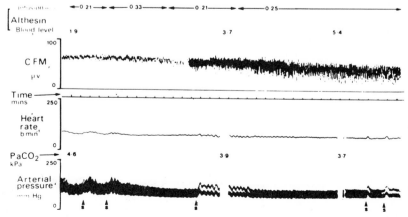

Figure 3. Response to stimuli in the presence of repeated small doses of fentanyl.

suggesting that cortical depression was increasing throughout the period. The blood level of althesin rose at the same time. A trace of pulse rate and blood pressure during the superficial phase of anaesthesia showed a variation in instantaneous rate and pressure. Stimuli applied over the tibia produced peaks in blood pressure and pulse rate (Fig. 3).

As this patient became more deeply anaesthetized, blood pressure and heart rate were slightly less variable, but another stimulus again produced a marked increase in both. For some reason the blood pressure continued to vary for some minutes, almost as though the autonomic nervous system had been woken up. It then went back to a smooth trace. Anaesthesia became deeper from the cortical point of view, but further stimulation still produced an increase in blood pressure and an increase in pulse rate. Finally we administered one small dose of fentanyl and 5 min later the response was reduced. At present one cannot be certain that these responses can be quantified. It is possible that they should be assessed either as present or absent.

In another patient anaesthetized in a similar manner and showing moderately deep cortical anaesthesia, noxious stimuli also produced reflex changes in blood pressure and pulse rate. Nitrous oxide was then given on the grounds that it is a standard anaesthetic and a good analgesic. But 10 min after the continuous ad-

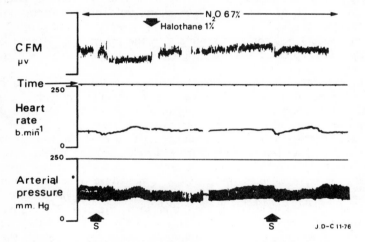

Figure 4. Response to stimuli in the presence of nitrous oxide.

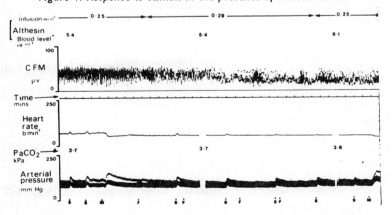

Figure 5. Response to stimuli in the presence of regular doses of fentanyl.

ministration of 67 % nitrous oxide the stimulus again produced rises in blood pressure and heart rate suggesting that nitrous oxide was not preventing the response (Fig. 4).

Figure 5 shows a trace from a patient given two initial stimuli which produced a rise in blood pressure and pulse rate. One mg of methoxamine was then given to check that peripheral vessels could constrict. There was a rise in blood pressure and a fall in heart rate suggesting that the baroreceptors were also working. We then gave four doses of fentanyl (0·1 mg) at 5 min intervals and stimulated the patient just before giving the next dose. In each case there was a rise in blood pressure and heart rate although it seemed as though the response diminished with successive doses. At the end, methoxamine was administered again and resulted in a rise of blood pressure which was broadly comparable to the original rise and a fall in heart rate, showing that the baroreceptors still seemed to be working.

In Fig. 6 the level of cortical activity was gradually increasing during most of the

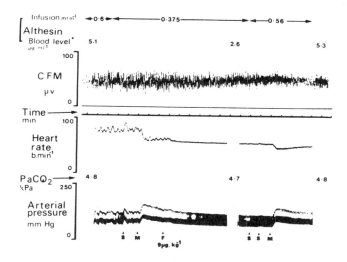

Figure 6. Response to stimuli following a single medium dose (9 μg/kg) of fentanyl.

study period. A noxious stimulus produced an increase in blood pressure and pulse rate and methoxamine produced an increase in blood pressure and a fall in pulse rate. A medium sized dose of fentanyl (9μg/kg) changed the character of the pulse rate and blood pressure making them less variable. Some 5 min later stimulation produced a barely perceptible response in blood pressure and heart rate. However, methoxamine still constricted peripheral vessels and reduced heart rate, suggesting that fentanyl was not having a direct peripheral vascular effect but was in some way preventing or reducing the response to noxious stimulation.

With fentanyl doses in the medium range (12 μg/kg) on average the rise in blood pressure is always reduced after fentanyl and in some cases it is almost completely eliminated. The increase in pulse rate is also always reduced. On the other hand, the percentage change in blood pressure and pulse rate due to methoxamine before and after fentanyl is similar.

Althesin anaesthesia might be considered unconventional so we have now started to study responses in patients anaesthetized with nitrous oxide, relaxed with pancuronium and ventilated to keep the $PaCO_2$ approximately normal. An example of

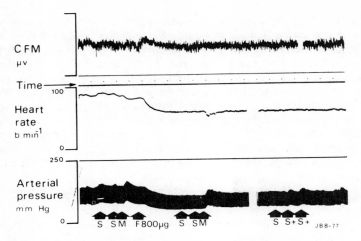

Figure 7. Response to stimuli following nitrous oxide and a single medium dose (800 μg) of fentanyl.

the typical response is shown in Fig. 7. Stimulation resulted in a rise in blood pressure and pulse rate whereas methoxamine produced an increase in blood pressure and a fall in heart rate (Fig. 7). Fentanyl (800 μg) smoothed the trace and little change in blood pressure or pulse rate could be detected following stimulation 5 min later. Methoxamine again produced a rise in blood pressure and a fall in pulse rate. After 8 min we applied the stimulus again and could not obtain any response. We then applied greater pressure and succeeded in obtaining a response. Clearly it is a matter of titrating the dose against the stimulus. A very noxious stimulus may require a very much larger dose than a small stimulus and perhaps these artificial stimuli are small compared to those of surgery.

Thirty minutes after the last dose of fentanyl the patient was taken into the operating room. The stimulus of the towel clip being put on the skin by the surgeon produced a rise in blood pressure. The incision produced an increased variation in both blood pressure and pulse rate. The pulse rate never exceeded 84, so that the patient did not

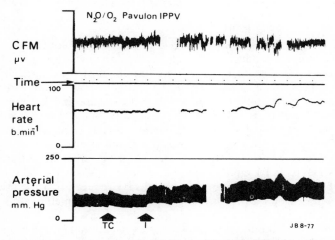

Figure 8. Response to towel clipping and incision following nitrous oxide and a single medium dose (800 μg) of fentanyl.

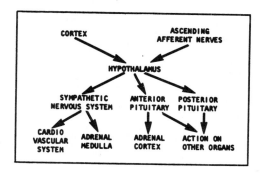

Figure 9. Components of the stress response.

have tachycardia. But the variation is very obvious compared to his previous condition (Fig. 8).

Three findings seem to emerge from these early studies. A drug like Althesin used to depress the cortex will not necessarily reduce the autonomic or cardiovascular response to a noxious stimulus. Attempts to reduce their effects with Althesin is therefore inappropriate and will not improve the quality of anaesthesia, merely prolong the recovery time. Secondly, fentanyl seems to be able to reduce the cardiovascular system response, even when the cortical activity is increasing. This confirms the notion that different anaesthetics act in different places in the central nervous system. It might be appropriate to monitor different parts of the central nervous system and then to give drugs according to the changes that are recorded. Finally it suggests that under the circumstances of this study variations in pulse rate and blood pressure seem to be increased with stimulation and to be reduced by narcotic analgesics, although hypertension and tachycardia do not necessarily result from such stimulation. This leads one to wonder whether it might be possible to monitor cardiovascular reflex responses more effectively by continuously monitoring variations in pulse rate rather than by intermittent measurement.

Table 1
Possible adverse effects of stress

Cardiovascular
    Increased heart work—tachycardia
                                —hypertension
        Dysrhythmias
        Vasoconstriction   —tissue hypoxia and acidosis
Metabolic
        Increased protein catabolism—impaired tissue repair
        Hyperglycaemia
        Reduced insulin secretion (initially)
        Sodium and water retention
        Increased potassium ions
        Increased mobilization and metabolism of fat—
            ?increased risk of thrombus formation
            increased ketone production
Depressed protection against infection and tumour growth
        Depressed inflammatory response
        Depressed immune response

Presumably these cardiovascular reflexes are part of the stress response (Fig. 9) and it is likely that they are signs that the patient is being stressed. Cardiovascular responses to noxious stimulation therefore suggest that the reflex arc is open and if the stimulus persists, then we think it is possible that the patient will experience all the signs of the stress response. A simple measurement of variation in heart rate might give some indication of the level of stress. For many years it has been believed that stress is a vital protective mechanism. Recently the protective importance of stress has been questioned. For instance, a number of anaesthetic techniques can reduce or even eliminate it without evidently harming the patient and an increasing amount of literature suggests that stress adversely affects a patient in a hospital environment.

Table 1 is a list of some of the suggested adverse effects of stress. Time will tell whether these effects are actually harmful and whether morbidity or mortality of patients is increased because they are being stressed. In the meantime, I think it appropriate that anaesthetists look for anaesthetic techniques which not only keep the patient unconscious but also reduce the stream of afferent impulses which evidently are pouring up the central nervous system during anaesthesia.

Analgesia and the Metabolic Response to Surgery

G. M. HALL

Department of Anaesthetics, Hammersmith Hospital, London, UK

The supplementation of nitrous oxide and oxygen anaesthesia with intravenous analgesic drugs, as opposed to volatile inhalation agents, is a superficially attractive technique. Unfortunately, the objective data to support the use of i.v. analgesics is in my view, weak, though elimination of the potent volatile agent certainly reduces pollution of the operating theatre and secondly avoids the occasional fatal toxic response to the volatile agent, such as malignant hyperthermia.

The arguments put forward for the use of i.v. analgesic agents during anaesthesia are based on grounds of cardiovascular stability such as Dr Savege has just described and also on a prolonged post-operative period of analgesia. However, nearly 20 years ago it was suggested that this prolonged post-operative analgesia was related to the fact that the patients were drowsy. On being awakened they still complained of pain.

My particular problem was to establish suitable anaesthetic techniques for use during Fallopian tube reconstruction. In a preliminary study using fentanyl in an incremental dose, which gave a total dose throughout 3 h of anaesthesia of 10 μg/kg, we found that the hypoglycaemic response to surgery was slightly reduced. We therefore performed a further study to investigate whether a larger dose of fentanyl namely 50 μg/kg had a significant effect on the metabolic changes during surgery and compared the results with those from a halothane control group.

Patients were premedicated with hyoscine and papaveretum. They were induced with thiopentone, intubated with the aid of pancuronium and maintained with nitrous oxide and oxygen supplemented with either 0·5–1·0% halothane or a bolus dose of 50 μg/kg of fentanyl given rapidly at induction of anaesthesia. We monitored the end tidal CO_2 concentration as in any metabolic study it is vital, in my opinion, to ensure that no hyperventilation is present. Core and skin temperatures were measured, together with blood pressure and heart rate determined by auscultation. For intravenous fluids, Hartmann's solution was used throughout.

Substrates assayed were glucose, free fatty acids, glycerol, beta-hydroxybutate, acetoacetate, lactate and pyruvate, and cortisol and growth hormone concentrations were also determined.

There were 13 patients in the fentanyl group and 14 in the halothane group (Table

Stress-free Anaesthesia: Royal Society of Medicine International Congress and Symposium Series No. 3, published jointly by Academic Press Inc. (London) Ltd., and the Royal Society of Medicine.

Table 1
Pre-operative patient data

	Fentanyl group (mean ±s.e.)	Halothane group (mean ±s.e.)
No. of patients	13	14
Age (years)	30·5 ± 0·9	30·9 ± 1·1
Weight (kg)	62·3 ± 3·4	56·6 ± 2·4
Body fat (%)	28·2 ± 1·4	27·6 ± 1·0
Duration of pre-operative starvation (h)	14·3 ± 0·8	13·9 ± 0·8

1). The groups were comparable in terms of age, weight, body fat and duration of pre-operative starvation. These latter two factors are of crucial importance when studying metabolism during anaesthesia, though in most cases they have been ignored.

With the induction of anaesthesia there was a significant decrease in plasma free fatty acid levels in both groups of patients, followed by a small rise. But at no time during surgery did the plasma free fatty acid levels reach pre-induction values. Glycerol concentrations had a similar trend. Many authors have suggested the use of plasma free fatty acid levels as an index of stress, lipolysis being particularly sensitive to the beta-adrenergic effects of noradrenaline. If this hypothesis is accepted, then these patients would appear to be more stressed in the anaesthetic room with the prospect of induction of anaesthesia and surgery than they were at any time during the surgical procedure. Ketone bodies showed a small rise during anaesthesia, but there was no significant difference between halothane patients and the fentanyl group in plasma free fatty acids, glycerol or ketone body levels.

However, blood glucose levels in halothane patients showed a rise of about 1 mmol/litre in the first hour of anaesthesia which was maintained for 3 h, whereas the fentanyl group showed no significant change in their blood glucose concentrations (Fig. 1). The plasma lactate in the halothane patients showed a significant rise during surgery whereas this was not present in the fentanyl group (Fig. 2). It is not clear why this significant, although numerically small, rise in lactate concentration occurred. It is often stated that by avoiding hyperventilation (which we most certainly did) there will be no significant change in lactate values. Many explanations have been offered and I would like to add one more. An increase in lactate concentration may be another indicator of the metabolic response to surgical stress. Similar findings

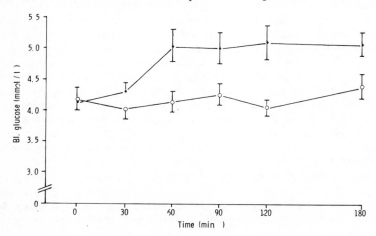

Figure 1. Blood glucose changes in patients receiving fentanyl (○) and halothane (●).

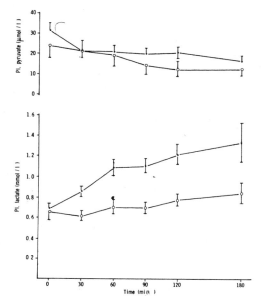

*Figure 2. Plasma, lactate and pyruvate in patients receiving fentanyl (○)
and halothane (●).*

have recently been made in burns patients. Differences in pyruvate levels between the
two groups were not significant.

The halothane group of patients showed roughly a four-fold increase in cortisol
levels during anaesthesia compared to pre-induction values (Fig. 3). The fentanyl

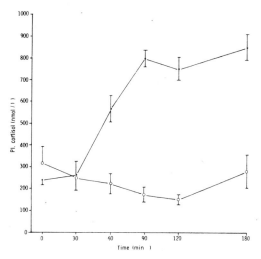

Figure 3. Cortisol levels in patients receiving fentanyl (○) and halothane (●).

patients, on the other hand, showed a decline in cortisol values and after 2 h the
difference from the pre-induction value was just statistically significant. There was a
trend back towards the induction values after 3 h. With growth hormone values the

variation was considerably greater. Nonetheless, the halothane group showed a rise in growth hormone concentration which was largely absent in the fentanyl group.

In conclusion, it would appear that for this particular duration of surgery and degree of surgical stimulation, 50 μg/kg of fentanyl completely abolishes the hyperglycaemic response, the cortisol response and the growth hormone response. It is likely that a lower dose of fentanyl (30–40 μg/kg) would have the same effect. Following this initial study, there were no post-operative problems. We have subsequently performed nearly 50 cases with a similar technique. There were two cases of apnoea in the recovery room within 10 min of completion and one case of delayed hypoventilation occurring on the ward 3 h after the finish of surgery. On the other hand, we have successfully established spontaneous respiration after 1·75 h of surgery with this dose of fentanyl.

The study raises several questions. For example, what is the survival value of the cortisol and growth hormone responses? In the fentanyl group, the plasma cortisol levels declined and some of the individual values were very low. And yet, from the cardiovascular point of view, as crudely measured by heart rate and blood pressure, the patient's condition remained stable.

Does this technique have any long-term value? I think it may be useful in trying to reduce the general catabolic response to severe trauma. If we can ablate the cortisol and growth hormone responses (and probably several other hormone changes too) it may be possible to decrease the catabolic phase in a patient admitted, for example, to the intensive care unit with major trauma. The other possible application seems to be in patients with disordered carbohydrate metabolism, particularly diabetics. The suitability of the techniques used for diabetics has never really been investigated. With this technique, in a diabetic patient at least, it might be possible to eliminate the surgical cause of changes in glucose metabolism.

Discussion

T. H. Stanley (*Salt Lake City*)

What was the duration of your operative procedure? Did you reverse the fentanyl activity in any of your patients and what was the average time for extubation or re-establishment of normal ventilation?

G. M. Hall

The duration of surgery was just in excess of 3 h. We did not administer naloxone in the initial series although we have subsequently done so. We have not measured the time taken to establish spontaneous respiration but my impression is that it is no longer than for any other patient who has just had 3 h of anaesthesia and surgery.

T. H. Stanley

Did you notice that any patients had prolonged respiratory depression?

G. M. Hall

The two that had apnoea in the recovery room appeared initially to breath adequately. Depression occurred within about 10 min of the end of surgery and I think that, providing adequate recovery facilities exist, this is not a major problem. Unlike the incremental technique, what you must not do with this method is give any more analgesic, otherwise there may be problems with establishing respiration post-operatively.

C. Conseiller (*Boulogne*)

It is difficult to understand the lactate responses in the absence of hyperventilation in the two groups.

G. M. Hall

The end tidal CO_2 levels were measured in both groups and they were the same, so I think it is reasonable to assume that there was not gross hyperventilation in the halothane group.

Attenuation of Stress and Haemodynamic Stability

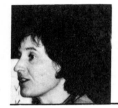

A. FLORENCE

Broadgreen Hospital, Liverpool, UK

My particular interest in the attenuation of "stress" is to maintain haemodynamic stability during major vascular surgery in patients who present with gross atherosclerosis. These patients are at risk of myocardial or cerebral damage in the presence of rapid fluctuations in blood pressure and pulse rate. They represent a group of patients difficult to study scientifically because they react abnormally to any form of "stress" response. In addition a vast number receive some form of adrenergic system blocking therapy in the pre-operative period in the management of hypertension or angina. The cardiovascular system is therefore severely compromised before any further anaesthetic or surgical insult is inflicted. To minimize depression of the myocardium or sudden change in the functional capacity of the vascular bed which would thus necessitate compensatory increase in the work of an ischaemic myocardium, I have been exploring the possibilities of using 25 μg/kg body weight of fentanyl as the primary anaesthetic agent. The patient is preoxygenated and an intravenous infusion established before fentanyl is administered over a period of 3 min. At the onset of apnoea, assistance is given to ventilation, and 80% nitrous oxide introduced. On disappearance of eyelash or corneal reflexes a non-depolarizing muscle relaxant—alcuronium 20 mg or pancuronium 8 mg—is injected. During the course of anaesthesia an increment of one quarter of the initial dose of fentanyl is given routinely at 60 min intervals unless it is required earlier, as indicated by either an increase in arterial blood pressure or, more frequently, pulse rate. All subsequent increments are then given at the same time interval, with the last administered not less than 30 min before conclusion of surgery.

With 25 μg/kg fentanyl a period of cardiovascular instability may occur at induction. This may be the result of the introduction of 80% nitrous oxide (Eisele *et al.*, 1976). In no patient receiving 25 μg/kg was there a hypertensive response to laryngoscopy; an increase in arterial pressure and pulse rate occurred at incision 20 to 30 min after induction, at a time of lessening analgesia; 5 to 10 μg/kg at this stage produced a stable state.

Haemodynamic stability was readily achieved with 25 μg/kg fentanyl during peripheral vessel surgery but not during aortic surgery. Significant hypertension was, however, not seen during dissection of the aorta and application of the occlusion

Stress-free Anaesthesia: Royal Society of Medicine International Congress and Symposium Series No. 3, published jointly by Academic Press Inc. (London) Ltd., and the Royal Society of Medicine.

clamp. The finding of no significant increase in either plasma adrenaline or nor-adrenaline suggests suppression of catecholamine release at this point (Au *et al.*, 1977).

Unlike Dr Hall I have found that lower dose levels of fentanyl do not suppress the hyperglycaemic response to major surgery. Blood glucose levels did rise significantly but the actual pattern of increase was altered. The period of occurrence of maximum increase being delayed with progressively higher doses of fentanyl from 10 to 25 μg/kg. In the small number of patients studied to date, neither noradrenaline nor adrenaline levels are significantly increased in association with changes in haemo-dynamic stability, suggesting that it is suppression of response to, rather than release of catecholamines which confers the property of haemodynamic stability on fentanyl. In this group of patients, cortisol levels were not significantly suppressed at the point of blood sampling. It would therefore appear that 25 μg/kg fentanyl does not suppress hormonal or metabolic response, nor does it ensure haemodynamic stability during major vascular surgery, where stimulation of the autonomic nervous system is frequently excessive.

References

Eisele, J. H., Reitan, J. A., Rashid, A. M., Zelis, R. F. and Miller, R. D. (1976). *Anesthesiology* **44**, 16.

Au, A. S. W., Evans, D., Crago, R. and Jones, W. M. (1977). *Canadian Anaesthetists Society Journal* **24**, 263.

Discussion

M. Zindler (*Dusseldorf*)

Clamping the aorta did not cause a rise in pressure. Was this a typical or exceptional finding?

A. Florence

Since I started using high doses of fentanyl, in about 95 % of cases, I see no hypertension at that particular moment.

M. Zindler

We must have different patients.

A. Florence

The policy that we have adopted is not to dehydrate these patients. We probably overload them in a determined effort to keep them excreting urine at a rate of approximately 600 ml/h. An average 70 kg man will receive about 600 ml/h of Hartman's solution so that the hypotension is not due to the fact that they are hypovolaemic.

Recently, a Canadian report suggested that the response was associated with an increase in plasma catecholamines. Unfortunately I do not have the plasma catecholamine levels of the current series, but in patients given phenoperidine, there was no increase in plasma catecholamines at the point of aortic handling and application of the clamp.

D. Kettler (*Goettingen*)

Have you seen any hypertensive crises and if one occurs and you then use a large dose of additional fentanyl, will it cope with the crisis?

A. Florence

Yes. Hypertensive crises certainly occur with much lower doses, for example 10 μg/kg, or using virtually homeopathic doses of phenoperidine. I saw them when using the "Liverpool technique" of anaesthesia, in which no analgesic was given and patients were hyperventilated to a paCO$_2$ of about 20–25 mmHg (2·6–3·3 kPa).

There are also problems in the post-operative period which have caused some concern. Three respiratory arrests have occurred, two associated with inadvertent administration of post-operative opiate when it was obviously not required; one occurred spontaneously. Blood gas estimations are made regularly at 30 min intervals. To our surprise we found that patients who had recovered spontaneously with normal tidal volumes at normal respiratory rates after reversal of the muscle relaxant, and in whom the respiratory pattern was maintained, were developing carbon dioxide levels of 60–82·5 mmHg (8–11 kPa) during the first 3–4 h post-operatively. At no time was this associated with hypertension, tachycardia or cardiac dysrhythmias, which one would expect with high carbon dioxide tensions. Arterial oxygen levels were maintained throughout within the range 110–150 mmHg (15–20 kPa). Apart from drowsiness there was no clinical necessity for IPPV. Within 3–4 h all patients were fully awake with blood gases within normal limits. Presumably hypercarbia was the result of alteration of the normal response to carbon dioxide in the presence of increased production of carbon dioxide. All patients became moderately hypothermic after prolonged anaesthesia with moderately high dose fentanyl, with the result that shivering and consequently increased carbon dioxide production is frequent in the post-operative period.

T. H. Stanley (*Salt Lake City*)

What is your criterion for mechanical ventilation after operation?

A. Florence

To avoid it as much as possible. This is because the surgeons with whom I work do not like automatic ventilators. But if we intend to use these doses of fentanyl, we shall have to think in terms of ventilating patients.

Fentanyl-Oxygen Anaesthesia for Patients with Mitral Valve Disease

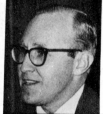

T. H. STANLEY and L. R. WEBSTER

Department of Anesthesiology, University of Utah
College of Medicine, Salt Lake City, USA

Fentanyl, in doses of 10 μg/kg produces little circulatory changes in man (Stoelting et al., 1975) and in doses of 20 μg/kg, little effect on left ventricular dynamics in blood-perfused dog hearts (Freye, 1974; Ostheimer et al., 1975). Large doses of fentanyl (0·05–2·0 mg/kg) plus oxygen result in little alteration of circulatory dynamics in the intact dog and produce adequate anaesthesia for thoracotomy (Liu et al., 1976). On the basis of these studies, we and a number of other clinicians have been routinely using high dose (50–100 μg/kg) fentanyl and oxygen or fentanyl, diazepam and oxygen as *complete* anaesthetics in open-heart operations. However, the cardiovascular effects of these large doses of fentanyl have not been investigated in man. In this study we measured the cardiovascular effects of anaesthetic doses of fentanyl (up to 50 μg/kg) during oxygen breathing and 50 μg/kg of fentanyl plus 10 mg of diazepam in 23 patients about to undergo mitral valvular replacement operations.

Patients and Methods

Written informed consent was obtained from each of the patients at the time of the pre-operative visit. All patients were premedicated with i.m. pentobarbital (60–100 mg) and atropine (0·3–0·5 mg), 90 min before the scheduled operation.

Prior to anaesthesia, an intravenous line was started in an upper extremity. A central venous pressure catheter was placed percutaneously into the right atrium from the antecubital fossa or neck and a radial or brachial artery catheter was inserted percutaneously and threaded 30–72 cm into the central aorta. The aortic pressure catheter was attached via an arterial pressure transducer to a central digital computer substation in the operating room. After appropriate calibration as previously described by Warner et al. (1968), his method of analysing the central aortic pulse-pressure curve was used to determine cardiac output, stroke volume, arterial blood pressure and peripheral arterial resistance.

With the patient breathing pure oxygen for a minimum of 15 min, fentanyl was

Stress-free Anaesthesia: Royal Society of Medicine International Congress and Symposium Series No. 3, published jointly by Academic Press Inc. (London) Ltd., and the Royal Society of Medicine.

administered i.v. at a rate of 50–100 μg/min for the first 4 min and 150–200 μg/min thereafter until the patients were unresponsive to verbal command and pin-prick stimulation. Respirations were first assisted and then controlled. Succinylcholine (1·5 mg/kg, i.v.) was then given and the trachea intubated. Respiration was controlled to maintain $PaCO_2$ (as measured in aortic blood every 15–30 min), between 30–35 torr. After intubation, additional fentanyl was administered at a rate of 150–200 μg/min until each patient had received 50 μg/kg. Following this, ten of the patients had diazepam (10 mg, i.v.) administered over a 20 sec period.

Cardiovascular data were recorded before and after 5 and 10 μg/kg of fentanyl and thereafter following every 10 μg/kg of the compound. Data were also recorded 2, 4, 6 and 8 min after diazepam. The surgical procedure began immediately after completion of the study. During operation, increments of pancuronium (1–3 mg, i.v.) were given as necessary. Additional fentanyl was administered at a rate of 200 μg/min whenever mean arterial blood pressure, heart rate or cardiac output increased 15% or more above pre-anaesthetic (control) values.

Results

The duration of operation was similar in the two groups, averaging 323 ± 37 min in patients receiving fentanyl only and 336 ± 41 min in patients receiving fentanyl and diazepam. Patients became unresponsive to verbal command and pin-prick stimulation after an average of 660 ± 189 μg or 11 ± 3 μg/kg of fentanyl (range 8–15 μg/kg). Administration of succinylcholine and intubation at this time did not significantly change any cardiovascular variable measured. Patients receiving fentanyl and oxygen alone required an average of 4510 ± 512 μg or 74 ± 10 μg/kg of fentanyl whilst those receiving fentanyl, diazepam and oxygen needed 4290 ± 441 μg/ or 69 ± 9 μg/kg of fentanyl for the entire operation.

Fentanyl (5 or 10 μg/kg) did not significantly change any cardiovascular variable studied (Table 1). Fentanyl (20 μg/kg) produced a significant reduction of heart rate and mean arterial blood pressure but did not significantly change stroke volume, cardiac output, central venous pressure or peripheral arterial resistance. Additional fentanyl, up to 50 μg/kg, did not further alter heart rate or arterial blood pressure nor change any other variable measured. Administration of diazepam after fentanyl decreased stroke volume, cardiac output, mean arterial blood pressure and peripheral arterial resistance and increased central venous pressure but did not alter heart rate. The latter changes were maximal 4 min after administration of diazepam but still present after 8 min.

No patient experienced chest wall rigidity nor were any difficult to ventilate at any time during anaesthetic induction or throughout the operative procedure. When questioned post-operatively, no patient experienced any pain during operation nor remembered any aspect of their tracheal intubation or operation.

Discussion

Large i.v. doses of morphine (0·5–3·0 mg/kg) plus oxygen produce little change in myocardial mechanics in isolated heart preparations nor in cardiovascular dynamics in intact, supine man (Flacke, 1968; Lowenstein et al., 1969). As a result, morphine has become popular as a supplementary or complete anaesthetic in patients with

Table 1
Cardiovascular effects of large doses of fentanyl and fentanyl plus diazepam (mean ± s.d.)

	Fentanyl dosage (μg/kg)							Time after 10 mg diazepam (min)			
	Control	5	10	20	30	40	50	2	4	6	8
Heart rate (beats/min)	67±8	63±7	59±7	55[a]±6	55[a]±6	57[a]±6	57[a]±7	59±8	60±8	59±7	58±8
Stroke volume (ml)	51±8	52±8	54±8	56±9	54±8	56±9	58±9	48[e]±6	46[e]±5	50[d]±6	51[d]±6
Cardiac output (litres/min)	3·4±0·5	3·3±0·5	3·2±0·4	3·1±0·4	3·0±0·4	3·2±0·5	3·4±0·4	2·8[ae]±0·3	2·7[ae]±0·3	2·9[d]±0·4	2·9[d]±0·4
Peripheral arterial resistance	23·8±1·2	22·7±1·1	22·5±1·1	22·0±1·1	22·0±1·1	21·8±1·2	21·2±1·2	20·3±1·2	18·1[bd]±1·3	18·6[bd]±1·2	19·1[bd]±1·2
Mean arterial pressure (torr)	89±8	83±9	80±8	78[a]±7	76[a]±7	78[a]±7	77[a]±8	69[bd]±9	61[ce]±8	66[bd]±7	67[cd]±8
Central venous pressure (torr)	6±2	5±2	5±2	6±2	7±2	7±2	7±2	11[ad]±2	11[ad]±2	11[ad]±2	10[ad]±2

[a] $P < 0.05$; [b] $P < 0.025$; [c] $P < 0.01$. Student's paired t-test compared to control values.
[d] $P < 0.05$; [e] $P < 0.025$. Student's paired t-test compared to values following 50 μg/kg fentanyl.

marginal cardiac reserve. Incomplete anaesthesia (Lowenstein, 1971), hypotension (Lowenstein, 1971; Arens *et al.*, 1972) increased blood requirements (Stanley *et al.*, 1974), antidiuresis (Mannheiner, 1971) and cardiovascular depression when combined with nitrous oxide (McDermott and Stanley, 1974) have been demonstrated as problems associated with morphine anaesthesia. Fentanyl produces little change in myocardial mechanics (Freye, 1974; Ostheimer *et al.*, 1975). Analgesic doses of fentanyl in man (10 μg/kg, Stoelting *et al.*, 1975) and anaesthetic doses in the dog (0·05–2·0 mg/kg, Liu *et al.*, 1976) cause minimal alterations in cardiovascular dynamics. As a result, large doses of fentanyl (as the sole anaesthetic) plus oxygen has been suggested as a good anaesthetic technique for patients with poor myocardial function (Liu *et al.*, 1976). However, the anaesthetic requirements and cardiovascular effects of fentanyl as the sole anaesthetic have not been carefully studied in man.

The results of this investigation demonstrate that 8–15 μg/kg of i.v. fentanyl when used as the sole anaesthetic produces unconsciousness and avoids any changes in cardiovascular dynamics during induction and intubation in patients with mitral valvular disease. The data also indicate that additional fentanyl, up to 50 μg/kg, results in small decreases in heart rate and arterial blood pressure but no significant changes in stroke volume, cardiac output or peripheral arterial resistance. However, addition of diazepam after large doses of fentanyl produces significant cardiovascular depression.

In a previous study in dogs, Liu *et al.* (1976) showed that the most significant alteration in cardiovascular dynamics produced by large doses of fentanyl was a reduction in heart rate. Similar, though less marked decreases in heart rate were found in this study. Liu (unpublished data) and Gardocki and Yelnosky (1964) have shown that bradycardia after fentanyl can be significantly decreased by premedication with atropine and totally abolished by surgical vagotomy. This suggests that, as with morphine, bradycardia after fentanyl is secondary to stimulation of the vagal nucleus in the medulla.

Atropine was used as a premedicant in this study. However, recent work in dogs and man (Liu and Stanley, unpublished data) suggests that slow administration of fentanyl, particularly during anaesthetic induction, can markedly reduce the degree of bradycardia in the absence of atropine premedication. Slow administration of fentanyl during anaesthetic induction also decreases the incidence of chest wall rigidity, a complication that was not seen in this study, but has been reported after fentanyl by Corseen *et al.* (1964).

Diazepam (5–10 mg) has little effect on cardiovascular dynamics in unanaesthetized patients with cardiac disease (Dalen *et al.*, 1969). Because of this and its well known amnesic effects, diazepam has been advocated as a supplement during anaesthetic techniques employing intravenous agents (Knapp and Dubow, 1970; Stanley *et al.*, 1976). In a previous report (Stanley *et al.*, 1976) we showed that diazepam (5 and 10 mg, i.v.) produced only modest decreases in heart rate and arterial blood pressure and a small increase in peripheral arterial resistance when administered after 2 mg/kg of morphine in patients with a variety of cardiac lesions about to undergo open-heart surgery. Depression of the cardiovascular system after diazepam was much more marked in this study.

Cardiac output and mean arterial blood pressure were reduced by 18 and 22% respectively when compared to control values and 18 and 10% when compared to values following 50 μg/kg of fentanyl. Since diazepam reduced stroke volume and peripheral arterial resistance and simultaneously increased central venous pressure, the data suggest that diazepam acts as a direct myocardial depressant when given after large doses of fentanyl.

In a group of patients similar to those studied in this investigation and also undergoing mitral valve operations, we showed that 1.5 ± 4 mg of morphine (as the sole anaesthetic) was required for the entire operation (Stanley *et al.*, 1975). In those patients, an average of 0.4 ± 0.2 mg/kg of morphine produced unconsciousness and less response to pin-prick stimulation. These data when compared to the findings in the present study suggest that fentanyl is 20–40 times as potent as morphine when used as a complete or sole anaesthetic.

In contrast to the patients receiving morphine for mitral valve operations, who had significant increases in heart rate and blood pressure on intubation, the patients receiving fentanyl in this study sustained no change in these or any other cardiovascular variables measured on intubation. Absence of change in cardiovascular dynamics, particularly of heart rate, in a patient with obstruction to ventricular filling is a desirable finding. However, it suggests that patients in the present study were more deeply anaesthetized than patients in the former study and that fentanyl, in anaesthetic doses, may be even more than 40 times as potent as morphine.

When used as the sole anaesthetic, morphine results in increased blood requirements during bypass, during the entire operation and for the first 24 h post-operatively (Stanley *et al.*, 1974). This has been attributed to the venodilating property of the compound and had been considered a serious disadvantage of morphine anaesthesia. Venodilation and increased blood requirements have not been noted after large doses of fentanyl (Stanley, unpublished). Indeed, there are some data which suggest that fentanyl increases venous tone and decreases venous compliance (Freye, 1977).

In conclusion, the findings in this study demonstrate that large doses of fentanyl (as the sole anaesthetic) with oxygen produce complete anaesthesia and minimal changes in cardiovascular dynamics in patients with mitral valvular disease. They also indicate that the addition of diazepam after large doses of fentanyl results in significant cardiovascular depression. The data suggest that fentanyl–oxygen anaesthesia may be an attractive alternative to morphine in patients with little cardiac reserve.

Summary

The cardiovascular effects of anaesthetic doses of intravenous fentanyl (up to 50 μg/kg) and similar doses of fentanyl plus diazepam (10 mg) were determined in 23 oxygen-breathing patients about to undergo mitral valvular replacement operations. Fentanyl was administered i.v. at 50–200 μg/min until the patients were unresponsive to verbal command or pin-prick stimulation. Succinylcholine was then administered, the trachea intubated, respirations controlled to maintain $PaCO_2$ between 30–35 torr and additional fentanyl given until each patient had received 50 μg/kg. Following this, 10 patients received diazepam (10 mg i.v.) over a 20 sec period. Cardiovascular data were recorded before and after every 10 μg/kg of fentanyl up to 50 μg/kg and 2, 4, 6 and 8 min after diazepam. During operation, additional fentanyl was administered whenever blood pressure or heart rate increased 15% or more above pre-anaesthetic values.

Unresponsiveness was achieved with an average of 11 ± 3 μg/kg of fentanyl. Patients receiving fentanyl alone requried 74 ± 10 μg/kg while those receiving fentanyl plus diazepam needed 69 ± 9 μg/kg of the former. Fentanyl (20 μg/kg) decreased heart rate and arterial blood pressure but did not significantly change stroke volume, cardiac output, central venous pressure or peripheral arterial resistance. Additional fentanyl did not further alter heart rate or arterial pressure not change any other variable measured. Addition of diazepam after fentanyl decreased stroke volume, cardiac output, blood pressure and peripheral resistance and increased central venous pressure but did not alter heart rate.

These data demonstrate that anaesthetic doses of fentanyl and oxygen produce minimal changes in cardiovascular dynamics but that addition of diazepam after large doses of fentanyl results in cardiovascular depression. The findings suggest that fentanyl-oxygen anaesthesia may be an attractive alternative to morphine anaesthesia in patients with little cardiac reserve.

References

Arens, J. F., Benbow, B. P. and Ochsner, J. L. (1972). *Anaesthesia and Analgesia* **51**, 901.
Corseen, G., Domino, E. F. and Sweet, R. B. (1964). *Anaesthesia and Analgesia* **43**, 748.
Dalen, J. E., Evans, G. L. and Banas, J. S. (1969). *Anesthesiology* **30**, 259.
Flacke, W. (1968). *Federation Proceedings* **24**, 613.
Freye, E. (1974). *Anaesthesia and Analgesia* **53**, 40.
Freye, E. (1977). *Arzneimittel-Forschung* **57**, 1037.
Gardocki, J. F. and Yelnosky, J. (1964). *Toxicology and Applied Pharmacology* **6**, 48.
Knapp, R. B. and Dubow, H. S. (1970). *Southern Medical Journal* **63**, 1451.
Liu, W. S., Bidwai, A. V. and Stanley, T. H. (1976). *Anaesthesia and Analgesia* **55**, 168.
Lowenstein, E. (1971). *Anesthesiology* **35**, 563.
Lowenstein, E., Hallowell, P. and Levine, F. H. (1969). *New England Journal of Medicine* **281**, 1389.
Mannheiner, W. H. (1971). *Southern Medical Journal* **64**, 1125.
McDermott, R. W. and Stanley, T. H. (1974). *Anesthesiology* **41**, 89.
Ostheimer, G. W., Shanahan, E. A. and Guyton, R. A. (1975). *Anesthesiology* **42**, 288.
Stanley, T. H., Gray, N. H. and Isern-Amaral, J. (1974). *Anesthesiology* **41**, 34.
Stanley, T. H., Isern-Amaral, J. and Lathrop, G. D. (1975). *Anaesthesia and Analgesia* **54**, 509.
Stanley, T. H., Bennett, G. M. and Loeser, E. A. (1976). *Anesthesiology* **44**, 255.
Stoelting, R. K., Gibbs, P. S. and Creasser, C. W. (1975). *Anesthesiology* **42**, 319.
Warner, H. R., Gardner, F. M. and Toronto, A. R. (1968). *Circulation* **38**, (Suppl. II) 68.

Discussion

O. Mayrhofer (*Vienna*)

When we were using the high dosage fentanyl technique in cardiac surgery about five years ago we noticed chest rigidity as well as abdominal rigidity with 50 μg/kg body weight. We were able to abolish that by using 25 μg/kg as the first bolus and then using 5–7 mg of pancuronium, after which we did not see it with the second dose of 25 μg/kg. Were you using a muscle relaxant?

T. H. Stanley

Once the patient was non-responsive, according to our criteria, we gave 10 μg/kg more before we attempted to intubate. We then used succinylcholine to intubate the patient and we continued our study without further relaxant up to 50 μg/kg. When the surgical procedure began, we then used pancuronium as a muscle relaxant. I believe the phenomenon called *chest* or *abdominal rigidity* occurs early and is related to the early speed of administration of fentanyl. We have seen it when we have administered fentanyl too rapidly. When we have been conservative and started very slowly, we have not seen it.

O. Mayrhofer

You did not mention antidotes. We have used naloxon routinely so that we were able to extubate immediately in about 50% of patients and leave them without post-operative ventilation.

T. H. Stanley

My impression is that routine use of narcotic antagonists after large doses of opiates is dangerous, because some patients become renarcotized. In addition, in patients with coronary artery disease, we have seen hypertension and tachycardia which is exactly what one is trying to avoid. So we do not use narcotic antagonists.

M. Zindler (*Dusseldorf*)

What is the duration of mitral and coronary surgery?

T. H. Stanley

The coronaries take about 6.5 h, the mitrals about 5.25 h. We ventilate them as long as they need to be ventilated, using our criteria. Extubation takes place on average at about 3–4 h. Sometimes the period is short, 1–2 h. Rarely is it longer than 8 h.

M. Zindler

Why do you use diazepam and not nitrous oxide?

T. H. Stanley

We used diazepam initially because we were not sure of obtaining complete anaesthesia. We do not use it at all now because we do not think it has any purpose. We do use nitrous oxide, in an interesting way. We have reversed the technique of using it as a primary agent with small quantities of opiate. Now, particularly in the coronary patients, after we have administered a large quantity of fentanyl and when we know that a stressful response is about to occur, we turn on 50% nitrous oxide for this stress, depressing the cardiovascular system, but also blocking the stress. When the stress has passed or the patient begins to tolerate it we turn off the nitrous oxide. Thus we have reversed the technique, using fentanyl with small quantities of nitrous oxide when needed.

C. Prys-Roberts (*Bristol*)

Have you quantified the blood pressure response to laryngoscopy and intubation in these patients after you have given them these large doses?

T. H. Stanley

Yes, there is no response, which implies that they do not become tachycardic, bradycardic or hypertensive.

Haemodynamic Influence in Deep Coma in Man of Equi-analgesic Doses of Morphine, Fentanyl and Sufentanyl

C. CONSEILLER and J. J. ROUBY

Hôpital Ambroise Paré, Boulogne-Billancourt, France

Several studies have been conducted on the haemodynamic effects of morphine and related drugs. It seems that such drugs act mainly by reducing central sympathetic tone. In order to establish the importance of direct myocardial and vascular effects, it seemed appropriate to study in individuals without sympathetic regulation (namely, individuals in cerebral death) the haemodynamic effects of fentanyl and sufentanyl at doses used for anaesthesia and to compare these effects with those of morphine at equi-analgesic doses.

Patients and Methods

Studies were made in eight patients, all of whom had a clinical history of cerebral trauma and were in coma. All patients were in a steady haemodynamic state without vasoactive drugs and remained in a steady state throughout the study.

Drugs diluted in 30 ml of saline were injected i.v. in a period of 3 min. The doses were: sufentanyl, $2 \mu g/kg$; fentanyl, $10 \mu g/kg$ and morphine 1 mg/kg. Three hours elapsed between the study of each drug in the same patient. Thus the study observed the effects, first of sufentanyl, then, 3 h later, of fentanyl and finally, again 3 h later the effects of morphine, all in the same patient.

Catheterization of right and left ventricles was performed and cardiac output was measured by thermodilution. For sufentanyl and fenatnyl data were recorded at the end of the injection and 3 min later. For morphine, data were recorded at the end of injection and 6 min later. Assessment of myocardial performance was made by pre-loading with 500 ml of the patient's own heparinized blood re-infused in 10 min in order to draw a left ventricular function curve.

Fentanyl had no effect at 3 min or 6 min on heart rate. By contrast, morphine and sufentanyl produced a fall in heart rate.

Stress-free Anaesthesia: Royal Society of Medicine International Congress and Symposium Series No. 3, published jointly by Academic Press Inc. (London) Ltd., and the Royal Society of Medicine.

Results (Table I)

Table 1

Haemodynamic changes following equi-analgesic doses of morphine, fentanyl and sufentanyl

	Sufentanyl		Fentanyl		Morphine	
	Time after starting injection					
	3 min	6 min	3 min	6 min	3 min	10 min
Heart rate	− 6[a]	− 9[a]	− 1	− 1	− 4	− 5[a]
Mean arterial pressure	− 7	− 9	+ 4	+ 3	− 4	− 1
Mean pulmonary artery pressure	+ 1	+ 4	+10[a]	+15[a]	+ 5	+14
Right atrial pressure	+ 4	+ 9	+21[a]	+29[a]	− 7	+14
Left ventricular end-diastolic pressure	+11	+11	+ 6	+14	+16[a]	+32[a]
Cardiac index	+ 1	− 1	− 1	− 1	+ 4	+ 6[a]
Systemic vascular resistances	− 7	− 8	+ 6	− 1	− 5	− 7[a]
Pulmonary vascular resistances	+ 1	+11	+24	+18	+ 5	− 9
Slope of left ventricular function curve (L.V.E.D.P. between 5 and 15 mm Hg)	−36%		−13%		−16%	

[a] $P < 0.05$
Doses: Fentanyl 10 μg/kg; sufentanyl 2 μg/kg; morphine 1 mg/kg.
Data are given in per cent of control values.

Unlike sufentanyl and morphine, fentanyl had no effect on mean arterial pressure. Unlike morphine, which elevated the cardiac index slightly, fentanyl and sufentanyl had no significant effect on the cardiac index.

Morphine and sufentanyl had a significant effect on systemic vascular resistance, but fentanyl in contrast had no effect on systemic vascular resistance at these doses. nor were the effects of the three drugs on pulmonary vascular resistance of significance.

Sufentanyl and fentanyl had a relatively marked effect on the right atrial pressure, but morphine had no significant effect on it. Morphine significantly elevated the pulmonary arterial pressure, but seemed to have no effect on mean arterial pulmonary pressure, perhaps because the cardiac index had fallen.

Fentanyl, sufentanyl and morphine had a significant effect on left ventricular and diastolic pressure. However, morphine and fentanyl had no effect on left ventricular stroke work index, although sufentanyl had a depressive effect. All three drugs diminish the slope of the left ventricular function curve, but fentanyl had perhaps a less significant effect than the other two drugs.

Discussion

In cerebral death in man, central sympathetic and parasympathetic tone is weak or absent. Thus one may assume that in the present study the haemodynamic effects of fentanyl, sufentanyl and morphine were due to a direct effect of the drug on the heart and vessels. Morphine and sufentanyl appear to exert a significant influence on systemic vascular resistance. By contrast, it appears that fentanyl in equi-analgesic doses does not act on resistance vessels in conditions of this study.

All three drugs significantly increase right and left filling pressure of the heart and pulmonary artery pressure. This increase in pulmonary and filling pressure is not surprising and the effect has been observed with morphine by several authors, in patients with coronary and valvular disease of the heart. An increase in filling pressure of the left ventricle not associated with change in stroke work index suggests a negative inotropic effect. The decrease in slope of left ventricular function curves further argues for a slight negative inotropic effect of fentanyl at these doses.

In conclusion, among the three narcotic drugs studied, it appears that fentanyl in man exerts the weakest direct chronotropic and inotropic effects. It does not exert any direct action on resistance vessels. The most potentially dangerous effect is perhaps the rise which it induces in cardiac filling pressure and pulmonary pressure.

Effects of Neuroleptanaesthesia on Haemodynamics and Post-operative Respiratory Functions in Patients Undergoing Minor and Major Vascular Surgery

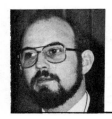

**H. J. WÜST, W. SANDMANN, O. RICHTER,
E. GODEHARDT and L. GÜNTHER**

*University Institute of Anaesthesiology and
Institutes of Biomathematics and Medical Documentation,
and Radiology, Dusseldorf, West Germany*

Patients undergoing elective vascular surgery on the abdominal aorta are classified as high risk patients because of a mortality rate of 6 to 15% (Lutz, 1967; Thompson, 1968; Vollmar, 1967; Wüst *et al.*, 1974, 1976, 1976a, b, 1977a, b, c). The risks are caused by three factors as listed below.

(1) Symptoms of arteriosclerotic disease. This is the most dominant risk factor. Hypertension, coronary vascular disease, myocardial infarction and a disturbed renal function should be mentioned. Furthermore the respiratory system is involved in every third patient (Thompson *et al.*, 1968; Wüst *et al.*, 1974, 1975).

(2) Cardiovascular disorders in many of these patients imply a decreased tolerance of the heart to acute changes in haemodynamics due to anaesthesia and surgical stimuli. Such changes are unavoidable because the aorta has to be clamped and declamped while reconstructing the arterial pathways. This can cause a cardiac failure by increasing the afterload of the heart or traumatic shock after the release of the aortal clamp (Attia *et al.*, 1976; van Ackern *et al.*, 1973).

(3) After upper abdominal surgery, respiratory disorders in the post-operative phase are seen more often than in other areas of operation (Simpson *et al.*, 1961; Beecher, 1933).

Neuroleptanaesthesia (NLA) is the anaesthetic method of choice for these patients because of the stability of the cardiovascular function under this anaesthetic regimen (Nobbe, 1976; Lutz, 1967; Gemperle, 1965). In our experience vascular patients become hypertensive following surgical stimulation (Wüst *et al.*, 1976b, 1977b). This may be due to surgery or clamping of the abdominal aorta. We therefore increased the dose of fentanyl given to our patients, but the higher dose can lead to

Stress-free Anaesthesia: Royal Society of Medicine International Congress and Symposium Series No. 3, published jointly by Academic Press Inc. (London) Ltd., and the Royal Society of Medicine.

post-operative respiratory problems, especially following major vascular surgery. To clarify this question we attempted to evaluate the haemodynamic response to anaesthesia and operation under neuroleptanaesthesia. The research was completed by a description of the post-operative cardiovascular and pulmonary situation following aorto-femoral bypass operations (AFB).

We studied nine patients undergoing saphena- and 23 patients undergoing aorto-femoral bypass operations, observing heart rate, aortic and right atrial pressure, and pressure in the pulmonary arteries and pulmonary capillaries. The cardiac output was taken by thermodilution. From the measured data it was possible to calculate the total peripheral resistance and the cardiac index. Furthermore the tensions of the O_2 and PCO_2 and acid base balance were measured prior, during and after operation up to the third post-operative day. Changes in the chest X-ray up to the third post-operative day were compared with the pre-operative status. The patients' age, duration of anaesthesia and the amounts of electrolytes and blood infused are shown in Table 1.

Table 1
Age, duration of anaesthesia and the amount of infusions given under the two types of operation

	Saphena-bypass	Aorto-femoral bypass
No. of patients	9	23
Age	50·2±11·5	59·3±9·3
Duration of anaesthetic (h)	4·8±1·1	5·5±1·0
Electrolyte infusion (ml)	2971±441	4059±1254
Blood infusion (ml)	—	2182±882

Anaesthetic Method

Neuroleptanaesthesia was applied as the classic type II with dehydrobenzperidol and fentanyl. Under the doses of dehydrobenzperidol and fentanyl the patients had no recollections of the operation, as we had observed in the early stages of the study using lower doses of fentanyl (Table 2). After an identical induction dose of fentanyl the demand of fentanyl was somewhat less under saphenous bypass operations than

Table 2
Doses of dehydrobenzperidol and fentanyl given to patients under saphena (S) and aorto-femoral bypass operations (AFB)

	Type of operation	No. of patients	DHBP μg/kg	mg	Fentanyl μg/kg	μg/kg/h
Induction dose	S	9	195·0±45·0	1·00±0·44	13·2±5·6	—
	AFB	23	180·0±20·0	0·91±0·27	13·0±3·5	—
Maintenance dose	S	9		1·84±0·84	25·8±15·8	5·20±2·90
	AFB	23		2·41±0·90	34·0±13·0	6·44±2·16
Total	S	9		2·83±1·06	38·9±17·8	7·90±3·10
	AFB	23		3·43±0·99	49·0±13·0	9·20±2·10

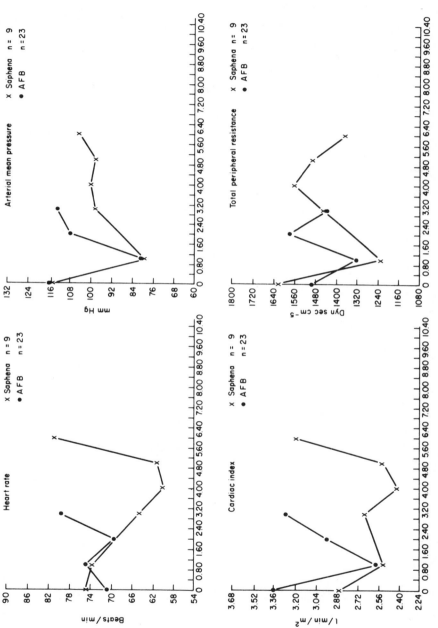

Figure 1. The response of heart rate, arterial mean pressure cardiac index and total peripheral resistance due to the induction of NLA type II in minor (saphena) and major (AFB) vascular surgical patients. Measurements were taken at: 0. = pre-operative control; 1. = just prior to the incision of the skin; 2.3.4. = 15, 30 and 60 min after the start of operation; 5.6. = prior and after 1 mg Atropine.

under AFB, as shown by blood pressure and heart rate response on operation. This was the case in relation both to the weight of the patients and the duration of anaesthesia.

The patients were artificially ventilated with 50 % nitrous oxide. The arterial PCO_2 was maintained between 35 and 42 torr. For post-operative pain release they were treated with continuous epidural analgesia.

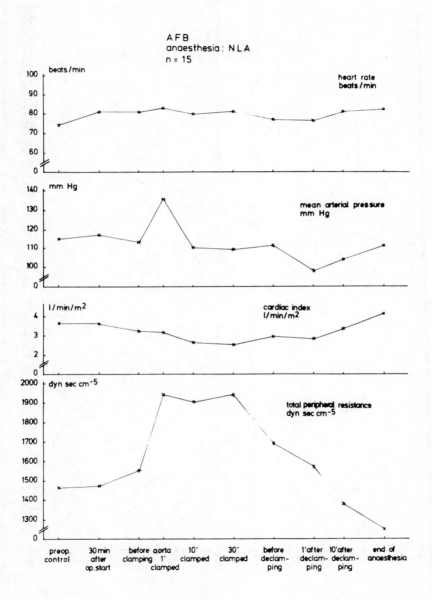

Figure 2. *Continued measurements of heart rate, arterial mean pressure, cardiac index and total peripheral resistance in 15 patients undergoing AFB operations.*

Induction of NLA and Start of Operation

Changes in the heart rate, mean arterial pressure, cardiac index and total peripheral resistance on induction of anaesthesia and the start of operation are shown (Fig. 1). The first point represents the pre-operative control, the second the status under anaesthesia just prior to the beginning of the operation. The next measurements were taken 15 and 30 min after the start of operation. The total peripheral resistance and mean arterial pressure decreased after induction of anaesthesia in both groups. In the AFB group the changes in mean arterial pressure were mainly caused by a 23% decrease of the cardiac index. The heart rate was slightly increased in the AFB patients receiving pancuronium. It was unchanged in the other group. Thirty minutes after the start of operation the total peripheral resistance and mean arterial pressure had almost increased to the pre-operative control level. Measurement of the vagal response showed a 46% increase in patients on saphenous bypass and a 26% increase in the AFB group.

Haemodynamic Effects of Clamping the Abdominal Aorta

The continued measurements of the cardiovascular parameters—heart rate, mean arterial pressure, cardiac index and total peripheral resistance in the 15 patients undergoing aorto-femoral bypass operation are shown in Fig. 2. Clamping the abdominal aorta increased total peripheral resistance, which lasted until the release of the clamps. There was an initial increase of the mean arterial pressure in three patients. In two patients clamping of the aorta caused a sharp drop of the mean arterial pressure. In one patient it fell from 90 to 60 torr, in the other from 90 to 32 torr. Five minutes after this procedure the blood pressure was lowered in the patients, having shown an increase, to the pre-clamp level. The cardiac index decreased by 21%. Declamping the aorta caused a decrease of the mean arterial pressure by lowering the total peripheral resistance and increasing the cardiac index.

Effects of Anaesthesia on Haemodynamics in the Post-operative Period

The effects of anaesthesia in the post-operative period up to the first post-operative day, under pain conditions and continuous thoraco-epidural anaesthesia on the heart rate, mean arterial pressure, cardiac index and total peripheral resistance after aorto-femoral bypass operations are shown in Fig. 3. In a randomized study these patients were anaesthetized either with NLA, halothane or thoraco-epidural anaesthesia. After the end of operation, all patients were treated with continuous epidural anaesthesia for post-operative pain release. No treatment was given unless requested, but 4–6 h after the end of NLA and epidural anaesthesia the patients asked spontaneously for pain treatment.

The cardiovascular parameters after epidural and halothane anaesthesia showed a sympathico-adrenal stimulation due to pain. After NLA the response was different. While the heart rate and mean pressure showed only a slight increase, the total peripheral resistance increased and the cardiac index decreased significantly. The start of the epidural anaesthesia lowered the total peripheral resistance and mean

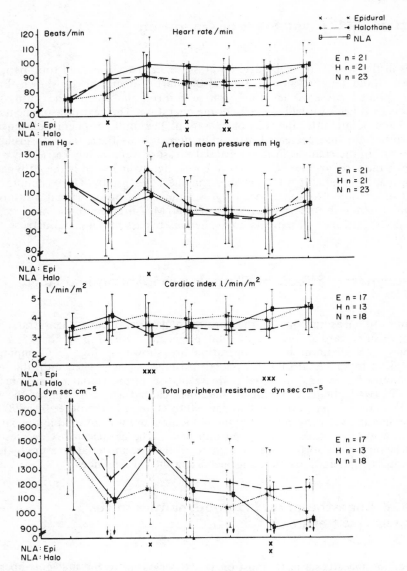

Figure 3. Influences of NLA II, halothane and thoraco-epidural anaesthesia on the responses of heart rate, arterial mean pressure, cardiac index and total peripheral resistance in the post-operative period due to pain and pain release by continuous thoraco-epidural anaesthesia. The patients underwent AFB operations. Significant differences between the groups were indicated by x at 5% level, xx at 1% level and xxx at 0·1% level.

arterial pressure in these patients. The cardiac index increased again. Compared with other groups, no differences except in the heart rate were found after the induction of epidural anaesthesia. This lowered peripheral resistance was maintained until the first post-operative day by means of epidural anaesthesia.

At the end of operation the arterial pH had decreased from 7·4 to 7·32, indicating a metabolic acidosis under NLA. This was intensified post-operatively for more than

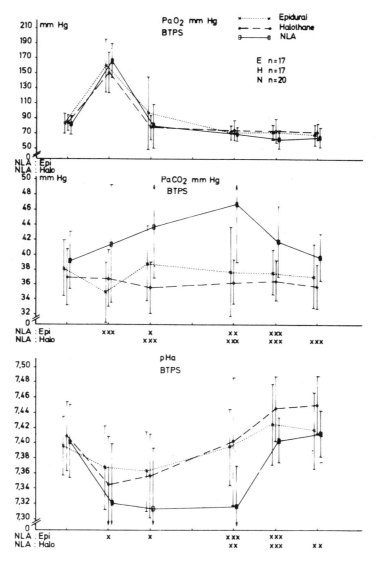

Figure 4. The influence of NLA, halothane and continuous thoraco-epidural anaesthesia on arterial PO₂, PCO₂ and pH. Measurements were taken 4–6 h post-operatively until the first post-operative day.

6 h by an elevation of the arterial PCO_2 (Fig. 4). In the other groups the changes showed a normalization of arterial pH after the start of epidural anaesthesia.

On the first post-operative day the arterial PCO_2 after NLA was within the normal range but still elevated in comparison to halothane and epidural anaesthesia. The changes of the arterial oxygen tension from the control to the first post-operative day are expressed as quotients. While the median of the quotient at the first post-operative day changed only little after epidural respiratory halothane anaesthesia, the quotient decreased after NLA by 28%. At the second post-operative day the quotient showed only a slight increase after NLA.

The PO$_2$ Q$_1$ quotient in the Wilcoxon-Mann-Whitney test indicate a significantly lower arterial PO$_2$ after NLA at the first post-operative day.

In 16 of 23 patients following NLA we found infiltrations in the chest X-ray. After halothane respiratory epidural anaesthesia only five patients showed pathological infiltrations in the chest X-ray. Until the third post-operative day there was only a slight increase in the rate of pathological findings.

Discussion

The data show that the blood pressure under neuroleptanaesthesia and operation is stable. Both in minor and major vascular surgery a stabilizing dose of 13 μg/kg fentanyl could not prevent reactions of the blood pressure and total peripheral resistance at the start of operation. These findings were in accordance with other reports, using only half or a third of the induction dose of fentanyl (Maunuksela, 1977). The response of the heart rate and cardiac index in patients undergoing aorto-femoral bypass operations shows the modifying effect of pancuronium (Kelman and Kennedy, 1971). Clamping the aorta led to an acute elevation of the total peripheral resistance related to an increase of the mean arterial pressure in 13 of 15 patients. This rise in the total peripheral resistance can cause an insufficiency of the left heart, as indicated by decreased pressures and cardiac index in our patients.

The total amount of 49 μg/kg of fentanyl had a significant influence post-operatively on the cardio-respiratory function, lasting at least 4–6 h. This may be the reason for a significantly higher incidence of hypoxaemia and infiltrations after NLA.

Conclusion

Patients undergoing minor and major vascular surgery in neuroleptanaesthesia type II showed an almost unchanged mean arterial pressure and total peripheral resistance during operation. But hypertensive reactions due to surgical stimuli could not be prevented by fentanyl in a total dose of 39 $\pm$ 17·8 resp. 49 $\pm$ 13 μg/kg. This amount of fentanyl caused a respiratory depression for more than 6 h after AFB operations and may therefore be the reason for the high incidence of post-operative pulmonary complications.

.

References

Attia, R. R., Murphy, J. D., Snider, M., Lappas, D. G., Darling, R. C. and Lowenstein, E. (1976). *Circulation* **53**, 961.

van Ackern, K., Brückner, K. B., Deuster, J. E., Reinberger, H. and Schmier, J. (1973). *European Surgical Research* **5**, 414.

Beecher, H. K. (1933). *Journal of Clinical Investigation* **12**, 651.

Gemperle, M., Moret, P. and Megevand. (1966). *Ann. Anaesth. Franc.* **7**, 87.

Kelman, G. R. and Kennedy, B. R. (1971). *British Journal of Anaesthesia* **43**, 335.

Lutz, H. (1967). *In:* "Anaesthesie in der Gefass- und Herzchirurgie." (Ed O. H. Just and M. Zindler) Anaesthesiologie und Wiederbelebung Bd. 20, Springer Verlag Berlin, Heidelberg, New York.

Lutz, H. and Müller, C. (1967). *In:* "Neuroleptanalgesie, Klinik und Fortschritte." Bericht über das III, Bremer NLA-Symposium am 21.u.22 Mai 1966. (Ed W. F. Henschen) pp. 107–118. FK Schattauer-Verlag, Stuttgart.

Maunuksela, E. L. (1977). *Acta anaesthesiologica Scandinavica*. Suppl. 65, p.1

Nobbe, F. and Dölp, R. (1976). *In:* "Der Risikopatient in der Anaesthesie" 1. Herzkreislauf-System. (Ed. F. W. Ahrefeld, H. Bergmann, C. Burri, W. Dick, M. Halmagyi and E. Rügheimer) Klinische Anaesthesiologie und Intensiv-therapie Bd.11, Springer Verlag Berlin, Heidelberg, New York.

Simpson, B. R., Parkhouse, J., Marshall, R. and Lambrechts, W. (1961) *British Journal of Anaesthesia* **33**, 628.

Thompson, J. E., Vollman, R. W., Austin, D. J. and Kartchner, M. M. (1968). *Annales of Surgery* **167**, 767.

Vollmar, J. (1967). "Rekonstruktive Chirurgie der Arterien," Georg Thieme Verlag, Stuttgart.

Wüst, H. J., Nadjmabadi, M. H., Sandmann, W. and Lennartz, H. (1974). Vortrag vor der Schwedischen Gesellschaft für Anaesthesie 28–30. Stockholm.

Wüst, H. J., Florack, G., Sandmann, W. and Lennartz, H. (1976a). *Langenbecks Arch. Chir.* **342**, S.594.

Wüst, H. J., Florack, G. and Sandmann, W. (1976b). *Exc. med. Intern. Congr. Series* **389**, S. 130.

Wüst, H. J., Trobisch, H., Godehardt, E., Günther, R. and Lennartz, H. (1977a). Vortrag auf dem 14. Kongress der Nordischen Gesellschaft für Anaesthesiologie, Uppsala.

Wüst, H. J., Sandmann, W., Florack, G. and Jesdinski, H. J. (1977b). Vortrag auf dem Zentraueropäischen Anaesthesie Kongress, Genf.

Wüst, H. J., Sandmann, W., Richter, O., Godehardt, E., Günther, R. (1977c). Vortrag auf dem 2. Berliner Lokalanaesthesie Symposium.

Discussion

T. H. Stanley (*Salt Lake City*)

You made the statement that you could not block the haemodynamic response at these doses. Do you think that you could by using a higher dose?

H. J. Wüst

We have not established that. We share the same problem as Dr Florence in that we have to extubate the patient at the end of the operation.

Stress in Neuroleptanaesthesia and Electrostimulation

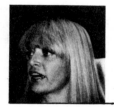

E. OTT and E. MARTIN

University Institute for Anaesthesiology, Munich, West Germany

The effect of electrostimulation versus fentanyl was investigated in a prospective double blind control study.

A group of 30 female patients undergoing elective gynaecological procedures was studied. In all patients anaesthesia was induced in the same conventional manner with valium, pentathol and continuous breathing of a nitrous oxide/oxygen mixture.

After induction but prior to surgery, acupuncture needles were inserted at four points of both ears and connected to an electrostimulator generating 12 mA and 60 Hz. A switch box, interposed between the patient and the electrostimulator, allowed transit or blockage of the electrical stimuli. The box was operated at random by a code which was unknown to both the anaesthetist and the surgeon throughout the study. Fentanyl administration was adjusted according to criteria which are given in Table 1. Wherever two out of the three haemodynamic or five vegetative criteria were

Table 1
Criteria for fentanyl administration

Haemodynamic		Vegetative
Increase of		Tears
heartrate	>25/min	Sweating
systolic BP	$>20\%$	Salivation
mean arterial		Colour of the skin
pressure	$>20\%$	Pupil reaction

At least two criteria had to be fulfilled for more than 3 min

present for at least 3 min, a single dose of 0·2 mg of fentanyl was administered i.v. During the whole procedure, arterial blood pressure and heart rate were continuously monitored. Only when all 30 patients had been investigated was the code opened. Seventeen patients were operated on during electrostimulation while the remaining 13 patients received none.

As far as the haemodynamic parameters are concerned, no difference was found between both groups for heart rate, systolic, diastolic and mean arterial pressure, until the end of operation. There was, however, a rise in heart rate and mean arterial

Stress-free Anaesthesia: Royal Society of Medicine International Congress and Symposium Series No. 3, published jointly by Academic Press Inc. (London) Ltd., and the Royal Society of Medicine.

pressure during extubation in the NLA group, probably as a result of increased sympathetic discharge.

There was no difference between groups in total consumption of valium, pentothal or pancuronium. However, fentanyl consumption was significantly lower in the stimulated group. Indeed, the total dose was only 5% of the fentanyl dose normally applied during neuroleptanaesthesia, 0·254 compared to 5·01 µg/kg/h. Thus, since the amount of conventional hypnotic necessary for induction of anaesthesia prior to operation was identical in both groups, the fentanyl saving in the stimulated group is probably due to the effectiveness of the electrostimulation *per se*.

In a second study of female patients undergoing gynaecological surgery we investigated stress factors. Neuroleptanaesthesia was performed with 5 mg of droperidol and 0·025 mg/kg of fentanyl. Electrostimulation was identical to that described above. In Figs 1–4 the abscissa refers to a control measurement in the conscious patient; 2 refers to the situation after induction and 7 and 8 refer to the first and second post-operative hour. Since the degree of dilution due to fluid administration was identical in both groups, the changes in concentration of different plasma factors cannot be explained by differences in blood dilution.

The mean plasma cortisol concentration rises significantly in the stimulated group

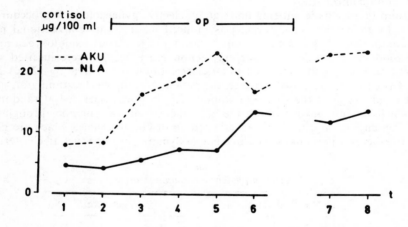

Figure 1. Plasma cortisol concentration in electrostimulation studies.

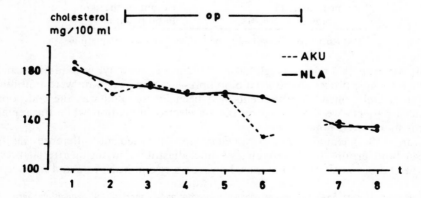

Figure 2. Plasma cholesterol concentration in electrostimulation studies.

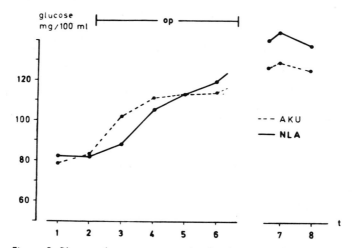

Figure 3. Plasma glucose concentration in electrostimulation studies.

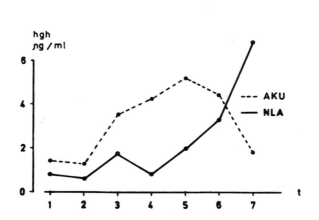

Figure 4. Plasma growth hormone concentration in electrostimulation studies.

after induction, stimulation and operation (Fig. 1). This probably reflects the stress of stimulation of afferent fibres with 12 mA, in addition to the stress of operation. Cortisol remains elevated post-operatively and the half-life is about 90 min. In the neuroleptanalgesia group there is a slight decrease between 1 and 2, caused by the bolus injection of fentanyl. Later during surgery, it rises significantly, because of operative stress.

Cholesterol is a cortisol precursor. Its plasma concentration shows an initial decline in the stimulated groups (Fig. 2). Intra- and post-operatively there is no difference between groups. The glucose concentration is almost identical in both groups (Fig. 3).

The human growth hormone concentration differs widely from one individual to another and is also dependent upon the diurnal rhythm. Because of this variation, there is only one significant point of difference between groups. This is at the end of the operative period where growth hormone concentration was found to be significantly below the value obtained in the neuroleptanalgesia group (Fig. 4).

In conclusion, it may be said that neuroleptanalgesia as well as electrostimulation are capable of producing adequate analgesia during surgery. Sympathetic discharge is present in both methods but is of only moderate degree. For lengthy operations or critically ill patients, electrostimulation has advantages if it permits the amount of neuroleptic drug to be significantly decreased.

Analgesia and Muscle Relaxation

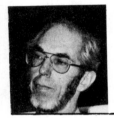

J. CRUL

Department of Anaesthesiology,
University of Nijmegen, Netherlands

I have only one simple point to make and that concerns the regaining of confidence in balanced anaesthesia. The necessity for adequate analgesia has been neglected for a long time in some areas of the world, particularly the Anglo-American anaesthesia area. An inborn resistance to intravenous anaesthetics was at the root of this behaviour and the claim was that it is much easier to reverse the side effects of inhalation anaesthetics because, by ventilation, they can be washed out, whereas the effects of intravenous drugs in the body are more difficult to reverse. In later years this was superimposed upon, and replaced by, the relaxant anaesthetic technique with hyperventilation of the Liverpool school, already mentioned in a previous page. There again, it was claimed that the hyperventilation increased analgesia and there was not a great need for analgesics to be added to the anaesthesia.

Under both of these conditions, the first with inhalation anaesthetics, the second with the hyperventilation technique, we still saw major stress reactions during painful periods of the operation. There was sweating, bradycardia and sometimes hypertensive periods. This, of course, improved considerably with the use of neuroleptanalgesia, practised for the last 10 years. I am certain that the criteria for adding or decreasing the amount of analgesics are just as specific as the indications for increasing the depth of general anaesthesia.

On the other hand, the role of muscle relaxants in balanced anaesthesia should not be neglected, even in this area of profound analgesia. Muscle relaxants have a margin of safety similar to or even greater than the analgesics. The reversibility of muscle relaxants is well understood and they can be handled well.

I claim that we should employ muscle relaxation liberally during these modern anaesthetic procedures with moderate or high doses of fentanyl, to avoid some of the major side effects of very high doses. Some of the signs of lack of analgesia are also signs which can be related to hypertonicity of muscle because of painful stimuli and reflexes to them. As such, they can just as well be abolished by muscle relaxants as by increasing the doses of analgesics. It is my belief that we should try to produce the same protection from stressful stimuli by increasing muscle relaxation as we do now by increasing doses of fentanyl. The same is true, I feel, for the hypnotic effect of some of the newer drugs that are now available in anaesthesia. Why should we try to induce unconsciousness and unawareness in our patients with very high doses of drugs which were not properly meant for hypnosis, such as narcotics?

Stress-free Anaesthesia: Royal Society of Medicine International Congress and Symposium Series No. 3,
published jointly by Academic Press Inc. (London) Ltd., and the Royal Society of Medicine.

The major interactions between the safe muscle relaxants and analgesics are minor, because they have different receptor sites and metabolic pathways. Therefore, the only potentiation occurs in the field of respiratory depression. Muscle relaxants can be more easily and effectively reversed than high doses of analgesics. We have studied the possible interactions on peripheral sites of action between high doses of narcotics and muscle relaxants and, like other authors, we found no potentiation of either drug by the other on neuro-muscular conduction. I therefore would suggest that we abolish autonomic stimulation to painful stimuli by the use of moderate doses of narcotics but we should not neglect muscle relaxation, so as to avoid some of the side effects occurring during anaesthesia.

Discussion
T. H. Stanley (*Salt Lake City*)

One of the advantages of fentanyl is its benignity on cardiovascular dynamics. However, the belief that if an agent is benign in itself then it will also be benign when added to another benign agent, is a very large assumption. For example, fentanyl plus nitrous oxide is not a very benign mixture and I think that your suggestion is valid only if the measurements are made which establish that a specific agent together with moderate doses of fentanyl produces a benign combination. It is wrong to make this assumption unless it is documented.

J. Crul

In the case of muscle relaxants, particularly the newer ones, such documentation exists for combination with analgesics.

T. Savege (*London*)

Apart from reducing oxygen consumption, what are the advantages which a muscle relaxant would have over an analgesic?

J. Crul

Holmes has pointed out, in his comparison of different anaesthetic techniques, that muscle movements can sometimes be signs of poor analgesia, reactions to surgical stimuli without being clearly painful reactions. Some of the increases in muscle tone are reflex mechanisms which do not go beyond the spinal reflexes and can much more easily be avoided or overcome by a muscle relaxant with its peripheral effect than by increasing doses of analgesics.

T. Savege

Alternatively, one may say that muscle relaxants disguise changes going on within a patient. By immobilizing him, one may think that he is well, when he is not. Such a situation may be dangerous.

J. Crul

I fully agree. First it is necessary to establish adequate analgesia. But who can give a clear indication of which doses are adequate?

R. S. Reneman (*Chairman*)

Professor Crul says that increased muscle tone can be abolished by muscle relaxants but I think that is largely the same way that fentanyl works. In other words, sufficiently high doses of fentanyl should be able to prevent hypertonicity due to pain stimuli.

J. Crul

We found that reflex increase in muscle tone after giving fentanyl can only be reduced by reasonably high doses of muscle relaxants.

Moderate Doses of Fentanyl by Infusion for Intraoperative Analgesia

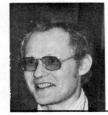

D. KETTLER and H. SONNTAG

Institute for Clinical Anaesthesia,
University of Goettingen, West Germany

Our group has for several years studied the effects of various anaesthetics on general and coronary haemodynamics, including myocardium oxygen consumption (MVO_2) and myocardial uptake of various substrates (Kettler, 1973; Kettler and Sonntag, 1974; Sonntag *et al.*, 1972). The general aim was to determine if there are anaesthetic techniques which are especially suitable for patients with coronary heart disease.

Coronary circulation is very sensitive to changes of haemodynamic variables, particularly heart rate, arterial blood pressure and inotropic state which typically occur during increase of sympathetic tone. Further indications of increased sympathetic tone are elevated arterial levels and increased myocardial uptake of the substrates glucose, lactate and free fatty acids.

Measurements were performed in patients scheduled for lung or vein surgery without evidence of other vascular or cardiac disease. All patients consented to participate in this investigation after being thoroughly informed of it's experimental nature. No premedication was given. Catheters were introduced into peripheral vessels under local anaesthesia and fluoroscopic control. Myocardial blood flow (MBF) was measured by means of the argon inert gas technique as described by Bretschneider *et al.* (1966) and Rau (1969). MVO_2 was calculated as: $MBF \times$ arterio-coronary venous O_2 difference. Effects of neuroleptanalgesia, applying droperidol and fentanyl, were studied as part of the general investigation.

On giving 25 mg of droperidol there was an increase of heart rate (HR), dp/dt_{max} and cardiac index (CI). Mean arterial blood pressure (MAP) fell slightly accompanied by a reduction of peripheral vascular resistance (PVR), (Tables 1 and 2). These haemodynamic changes produced a rise of MBF, MVO_2 and a reduction of coronary vascular resistance (CVR) (Table 2, Fig. 1).

From other studies (Whitwam and Russell, 1971; Yelnosky *et al.*, 1964) there is evidence that these changes are mainly due to an acute α-adrenergic blockade by droperidol and not to an increased β-stimulation. The subsequent injection of 0·5 mg fentanyl brought back all values to the awake status or even below.

Myocardial uptake of glucose, lactate, pyruvate and free fatty acids slightly increased under droperidol and again decreased under fentanyl (Fig. 2). However,

Stress-free Anaesthesia: Royal Society of Medicine International Congress and Symposium Series No. 3, published jointly by Academic Press Inc. (London) Ltd., and the Royal Society of Medicine.

Table 1
Haemodynamic effects of neuroleptanalgesia (NLA)—droperidol (DROP) and fentanyl (FE) in man

NLA (n = 10) DROP 0·33 mg/kg FE 0·0067 mg/kg	Before $\overline{x}$	DROP $\overline{x}$	DROP/FE $\overline{x}$
Heart rate (b/min)	77 ·	94[a]	79[a]
CI (l/min·m³)	3·72	3·93	3·43
SVI (ml/m³)	48	45	44
PVR $\left(\dfrac{mm\ Hg}{ml/min·kg}\right)$	0·99	0·84	0·98
MAP (mm Hg)	105	91	93
dp/dt_{max} (mm Hg/sec)	2260	2370[b]	2140[b]

[a] $P < 0.05$; [b] $P < 0.01$

CI	= cardiac index
SVI	= stroke volume index
PVR	= peripheral vascular resistance
MAP	= mean arterial pressure
dp/dt_{max}	= first derivative of left ventricular pressure

Table 2
Effects of neuroleptanalgesia (NLA)—droperidol (DROP) and fentanyl (FE)

NLA (n = 10) DROP 0·33 mg/kg FE 0·0067 mg/kg	Before $\overline{x}$	DROP $\overline{x}$	DROP/FE $\overline{x}$
MBF (ml/min·100 g)	97	139[c]	92[c]
CVR $\left(\dfrac{mm\ Hg}{ml/min.100\ g}\right)$	0·91	0·60[c]	0·93[c]
MADP (mm Hg)	92	86	86
MVO_2 (ml/min·100 g)	10·3	14·7[c]	9·2[c]
Hb (g%)	12·7	12·5	12·4
O_2-Sat. cor. ven. (%)	31·1	31·2	33·3
$avDO_2$ (Vol. %)	10·8	11·0	10·4

[c] $P < 0.005$

(FE)—on coronary haemodynamics in man	
MBF	= myocardial blood flow
CVR	= coronary vascular resistance
MADP	= mean arterial diastolic pressure (coronary perfusion pressure)
MVO_2	= myocardial oxygen consumption
·Hb	= haemoglobin content
O_2-Sat. cor. ven.	= coronary sinus O_2-saturation
$avDO_2$	= arterio-coronary sinus O_2-difference

these differences are not statistically different. Because of the results of this study and clinical experience we have abandoned droperidol at least in coronary risk patients. In other cases the dose is reduced to about 5–7·5 mg. However, the most striking improvement in analgesic technique was achieved several years ago when the method of incremental injections of fentanyl was changed to a continuous fentanyl

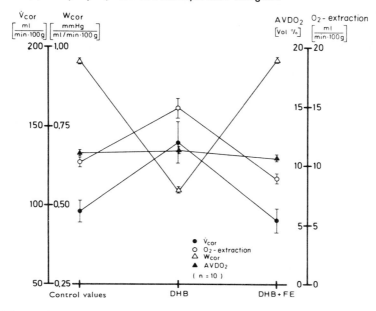

Figure 1. Effects of neuroleptanalgesia on coronary haemodynamics and myocardial O₂
consumption. V_{cor} = MBF; W_{cor} = CVR; AVDO₂ = *arterio-coronary sinus O₂-difference*
Control values (awake status); DHB = droperidol effects; DHB + FE = effects after additional
fentanyl injection.

infusion, controlled by an infusion pump (Staffregen *et al.*, 1972). Not only the level
of analgesia became more steady but the average dose of fentanyl could be reduced
also. At the present time we have observed about 100,000 cases of anaesthesia by
infusion analgesia.

In brief the technique is as follows: after premedication with 5 mg droperidol and
0·1 mg fentanyl, induction is performed with 1 mg/kg methohexital or 0·2 mg/kg
etomidate, the latter having only very little effect on respiration and circulation.
Before intubation the fentanyl drip containing 0·5 mg fentanyl in 250 ml electrolyte
solution or for longer lasting operations 1 mg fentanyl/500 ml is started. In the first
5 min 100 μg fentanyl are given and thereafter a continuous infusion ratio of 5–7
μg/kg/h is maintained using a constant volume infusion pump. Thus during a 3 h
operation, 15–20 μg/kg fentanyl are infused. Children need a higher dose of about
10 μg/kg/h. In addition, all patients are ventilated with nitrous oxide (50–70%) and
oxygen (50–30%). This, in comparison to Dr Stanley's technique, is a 3–4 times
lower dose of fentanyl and is, in our opinion, sufficient to produce adequate analgesia
during an operative procedure. It remains doubtful whether side effects such as hypertension, tachycardia and metabolic changes seen in a few cases should be solely
attributed to "stress" because of inadequate analgesia. Therefore, the question
arises whether it is wise to treat such occurrences simply by increasing the dose of
an analgesic drug to an undefinable level of analgesia. It must be borne in mind that
large doses of morphinomimetics have a strong hypnotic effect. But this part of
balanced anaesthesia can be better achieved with true hypnotic drugs such as benzo-
diazepines or steroid compounds. It should also be remembered that side effects of
morphinomimetics, particularly respiratory depression, bradycardia and increased
bronchomotor tone are dose dependent.

Whatever the philosophy of high or low doses of morphinomimetics it is necessary

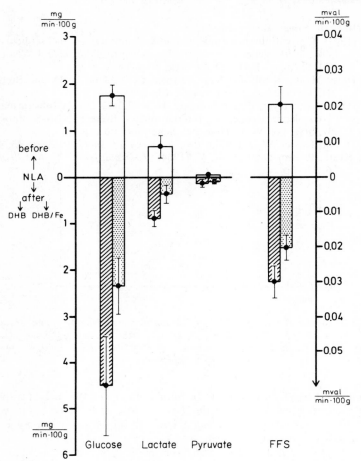

Figure 2. Effects of neuroleptanalgesia (NLA) on myocardial uptake of glucose, lactate, pyruvate and free fatty acids (FFS) in man. Measurements were performed before and after injection of droperidol (DHB) and additional fentanyl (DHB/FE).

to raise three questions. First, what do small changes in sympathetic tone and circulation during anaesthesia mean to the welfare of the patient? Secondly, should we use an analgesic drug only for analgesia or should we use it for anything else? And finally, should we treat certain occurrences during anaesthesia, such as hypertension, with specific drugs or always by increasing the dose of analgesic. We have to come to the point of having to decide.

References
Bretschneider, H. J., Cott, L., Hilgert, G., Probst, R. and Rau, G. (1966). *Verh. dtsch. Ges. Kreisl.-Forsch.* **32**, 267.
Kettler, D. (1973). Sauerstoffbedarf und Sauerstoffversorgung des Herzens in Narkose. Anaesthesiologie und Wiederbelebung 67. Springer, Berlin-Heidelberg, New York.
Kettler, D. and Sonntag, H. (1974). *Acta anaesthes. belg.* **25**, 384.

Rau, G. (1969). *Arch. Kreisl.-Forsch.* **58,** 322.

Sonntag, H. (1973). Coronardurchblutung und Energieumsatz des menschlichen Herzens unter verschiedenen Anaesthetica. Anaesthesiologie und Wiederbelebung 79. Springer, Berlin-Heidelberg, New York.

Sonntag, H., Heiss, H. W., Knoll, D., Regensburger, D., Schenk, H. D. and Bretschneider, H. J. (1972). *Z. Kreisl.-Forsch.* **61,** 1092.

Stoffregen, J., Opitz, A., Meyer, E. and Sonntag, H. (1972). Die NLA-Infisionsnarkose. *In:* Neuroleptanalgesie. V. Internationales Bremer NLA-Symposium, Teil II, hrsg. von W. F. Henschel. Schattauer, Stuttgart.

Whitwam, J. H. and Russel, W. J. (1971). *British Journal of Anaesthesiology* **43,** 481.

Yelnosky, J., Kratz, R. and Dietrich, E. V. (1964). *Toxicology and Applied Pharmacology* **6,** 37.

Effects of High Doses of Fentanyl in Comparison with Electrostimulation

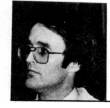

E. MARTIN and E. OTT

University Institute for Anaesthesiology, Munich, West Germany

The stability of the cardiovascular systems to high doses of fentanyl has been reported by many authors, especially in relation to high risk patients in cardiac surgery. Electrostimulation seems to be another technique for high risk patients. We have compared these two methods by measuring a number of haemodynamic parameters in 26 patients undergoing abdominal urological and lower abdominal surgical operations. Eleven patients were anaesthetized by electrostimulation; 15 patients received high doses of fentanyl. After premedication, (1·5–2 ml thalamonal+0·5 mg atropine), catheters were inserted and 10 min later systolic, diastolic and mean arterial pressure, cardiac output, heart rate, pulmonary arterial pressure, were measured, and stroke volume, cardiac index, right and left ventricular stroke work,

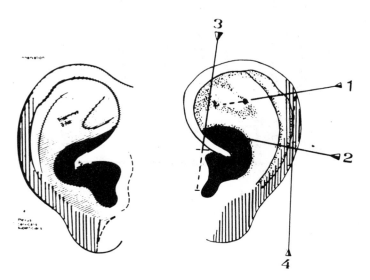

Figure 1. Position of acupuncture needles.

Stress-free Anaesthesia: Royal Society of Medicine International Congress and Symposium Series No. 3 published jointly by Academic Press Inc. (London) Ltd., and the Royal Society of Medicine.

pulmonary vascular resistance. total peripheral resistance and tension-time index were determined as control values.

Etomidate, 0·3 mg/kg body weight and succinylcholine, 1 mg/kg body weight were then administered, for induction of anaesthesia. Fentanyl 0·02 mg/kg body weight was also given to the patients in that group. Patients in the acupuncture group,·after the same induction procedure, received eight needles at four points in both ears (Fig. 1). The aim of this technique is to stimulate the areas innervated by the vagus and plexus cervicalis. These needles were connected to an electrostimulator generating 12 mA at 60 Hz.

In presenting the results, C indicates control values of conscious patients; NE indicates a time 10 min after induction. T_0 represents the beginning of the operation and T_1-T_4 are respectively 10, 40, 50 and 90 min after its onset. For the fentanyl group, T_2 is the period before the second dose of 0·02 mg/kg; T_3 and T_4 are 10 and 40 min later. T_5 represents the end of the operation and T_6 is 10 min after extubation.

After induction, there was a slight decrease in mean arterial pressure in the fentanyl group. In the acupuncture group, after induction there was a constant mean arterial pressure over the whole period of operation, with a significant rise only after extubation (Fig. 2) as well as in the fentanyl group. Cardiac index in the fentanyl group

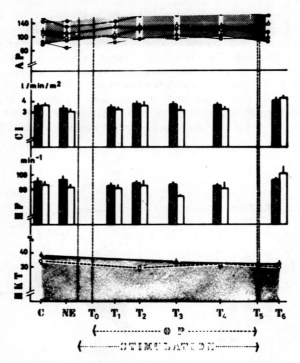

Figure 2. Heart rate, cardiac index and arterial pressure in fentanyl and acupuncture patients.

also showed a slight decrease after induction, but was largely constant so that there were no statistically significant differences in these two parameters between the two groups. The heart rate in the fentanyl group fell after induction and after the second dose of fentanyl there was no corresponding change in the mean arterial pressure.

Changes in pulmonary haemodynamic parameters were only significant after induction. During the whole period there were no significant differences in pulmonary vascular resistance or total peripheral resistance between the two groups.

Left ventricular stroke work in the two groups showed differences after induction. The decrease in the fentanyl group was much higher than in the acupuncture group (Fig. 3). During the operation there were no differences but after extubation there

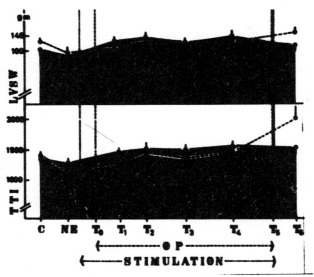

Figure 3. Left ventricular stroke work in fentanyl and acupuncture patients.

was an increase in this parameter, which was significant ($P<0.05$). The tension-time index showed the same behaviour in the two groups. There was only a significant rise after extubation.

In conclusion we have found that these two methods are capable of producing adequate analgesia, but electrostimulation had some advantages. Extubation occurs with a conscious cooperative patient. The anaesthetic demand is reduced under acupuncture and the demand for analgesic agents in the post-operative period is no higher than in the fentanyl group.

Discussion
O. Mayrhofer (*Vienna*)

> We have been using electrostimulation, with ear acupuncture needles but without fentanyl, in cardiac anaesthesia. And the longer the procedure, the better the analgesic effect. We have no proof about the degree of stress in comparison to other techniques but patients can be talked to during the procedure. They are fully awake as soon as we switch off the nitrous oxide/oxygen and yet they do not complain about pain post-operatively for some hours.

Analgesic Effects and Side Effects of Fentanyl in Man

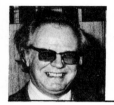

P. VIARS

Department of Anaesthesiology,
Hôpital Pitié Salpétrière, Paris, France

Fentanyl is accepted as being a potent analgesic, 75–300 times more potent than morphine and is generally believed to have a fairly short duration of action. However, many authors have observed quite a long lasting residual post-operative analgesia, although clinical conditions often do not allow satisfactory analysis of the various criteria of analgesia. It therefore seemed of interest to set up a study with no drug interference. The trial design consisted in acute administration to conscious volunteers of i.m. fentanyl citrate and morphine chlorhydrate in increasing dosages, the objective being to compare both products. Patients were assigned at random in groups of 10 each, according to the best available clinical criteria.

Table 1 shows the dosage ranges of both products administered in each series. The first group received a saline solution in order to establish any placebo effect. Table 2 shows the evaluation scale for analgesia. It should be noted that pain was tolerable but was perceived all the time.

Table 1
Doses of morphine chlorhydrate and fentanyl citrate

Substance administered	Dosage (μg/kg)
Normal saline	
Morphine	100
	150
	200
Fentanyl	1·5
	3·0
	6·0

Figure 1 shows the values of residual pain for each group after morphine and placebo. Analgesia increases in intensity and duration according to the administered dose. Figure 2 shows similar data for fentanyl, where the duration of action was longer

Stress-free Anaesthesia: Royal Society of Medicine International Congress and Symposium Series No. 3, published jointly by Academic Press Inc. (London) Ltd., and the Royal Society of Medicine.

Table 2
Clinical evaluation of pain

Rating	Description
5	Intolerable
4	Strong
3	Tolerable
2	Slight
1	Very slight
0	No pain

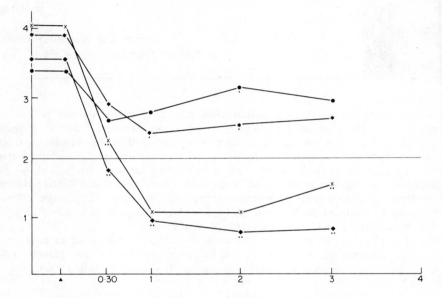

Figure 1. Variations in pain intensity after i.m. injection of morphine chlorhydrate.
Pain rating (ordinate) against time h (abscissa).

● Placebo
★ 100 μg/kg   ● P < 0·01
✕ 150 μg/kg
◆ 200 μg/kg   ●● P < 0·001

than expected. The range of equal activity lies at 0·15 mg/kg of morphine and 0·006 mg/kg of fentanyl, a ratio of 1:25.

The duration of clinically significant action increased for fentanyl with the dose, but did not differ from that of morphine at dosages of equal activity. Bradycardia, which was initially less apparent with fentanyl, became identical to that of morphine after 2 h. However, fentanyl did not induce hypotension. Respiratory depression at equal analgesic doses was equivalent for both products, but disappeared more rapidly with fentanyl. Subjective side effects for morphine were mainly numbness and nausea and for fentanyl slight euphoria and dizziness. Objective side effects such as sedation and drowsiness were equally shared by the two compounds, whereas such reactions as sweating and whiteness were more frequent with morphine.

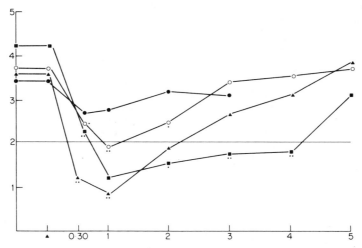

Figure 2. *Variations in pain intensity after i.m. injection of fentanyl citrate.*
Pain rating (ordinate) against time (h) (abscissa).

● Placebo
○ 1·5 µg/kg   ● $P < 0.01$
▲ 3·0 µg/kg
■ 6·0 µg/kg   ● ● $P < 0.001$

The conclusion of this study is that fentanyl citrate is a potent analgesic, 25 times more potent than morphine. At equi-analgesic dosages its profile of activity is quite similar to that of morphine. Side effects are also similar.

Discussion

D. Kettler (*Goettingen*)

That was a beautiful study, but I would like to ask if you have any explanation for the low potency ratio of 25:1 between fentanyl and morphine.

P. Viars

This study was free from outside drug influence whereas the other data published so far were obtained under clinical conditions with interactions between drugs and anaesthetics. In man, in the conscious state in this trial design, a ratio of 25:1 can be considered quite high. In eight other studies, analgesics have been compared under the same conditions and the ratios found here are consistent with the other published ratios.

R. Cookson (*Marlow*)

It is very difficult to compare two drugs which could have .different durations of action and to comment both on duration of action and on potency in the same study. Increasing the dosage of the shorter acting drug might produce a longer duration of action, and that might be one explanation for this lower ratio. Dundee and Clark used i.m. doses of 0·1 or 0·2 mg of fentanyl and 10 mg of morphine in conscious volunteers. Using their index of responses to somatic pain, fentanyl was active for about 20–25 min but morphine was completely inactive, which would suggest that the ratio is at least 50:1.

T. H. Stanley (*Salt Lake City*)

The ratio may also change depending on the dosage range, 25:1 at one range of dosages and 100:1 at another.

P. Viars

I agree with Dr Cookson that it is difficult to compare two rather different drugs, but since they are being used as reference compounds a comparison was needed and the study was warranted. I also agree with Dr Stanley but this is a problem with all comparative data in pharmacological studies.

The Use of Certain Morphinomimetics in Acute Clinical Situations

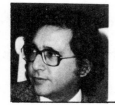

P. GLASER

Department of Anaesthesiology,
Hôpital Pitié Salpêtrière, Paris, France

Difficulty in the use of the ventilator, especially with some critically ill patients, is a situation which sometimes faces the anaesthetist in a surgical intensive care unit. However, it is important to bring patients in acute states under control, otherwise respiratory muscle work and oxygen consumption increase. We believe that morphinomimetic drugs have advantages in permitting adaptation to the ventilator, with very few side effects.

The purpose of this prospective study was to evaluate this belief for the long-acting morphinomimetic drug *piritramide*. The study involved five main considerations: rapid adaptation to the ventilator; sedation of restlessness; regard for a sufficient level of consciousness; duration of action of the drug and, finally, cardiovascular acceptability.

The clinical data were determined on 30 patients, 24 men and six women, average age 38 years. Indications for the drug were uncontrolled ventilation in all cases; restlessness in seven patients and acute post-operative pain in four. Intravenous injection of piritramide 15 mg was every 6 h, with re-injection when necessary. We observed the degree of sedation, adaptation to the ventilator and the level of consciousness at hourly intervals over a long time-course. We also tried to analyse any chronic symptom of intoxication, i.e. tolerance, addiction and withdrawal symptoms. The duration of the study varied from 8–26 days depending on the patient.

The average dose of piritramide per patient was 335·4 mg (range 45–1485 mg). The average dose/kg per injection was 0·23 mg (range 0·17–0·37).

Intravenous injection of 15 mg of piritramide produced an adequate level of sedation in 86% of cases. Adaptation to the ventilator was obtained in 81% of the cases. Sleepiness occurred, at one time or another, in 50% and about 10% lapsed into unconsciousness. These cases were not well selected for this drug. An i.v. dose of 15 mg produced an effect lasting from 1–6 h (mean, 198 minutes, or more than 3 h). Five patients showed tolerance to the drug after 4–12 days, having received 165–640 mg. Addiction was observed in only one patient on the eighteenth day with a total dosage of 1g. Withdrawal symptoms were observed in one case on the sixth day.

Stress-free Anaesthesia: Royal Society of Medicine International Congress and Symposium Series No. 3, published jointly by Academic Press Inc. (London) Ltd., and the Royal Society of Medicine.

We also performed some haemodynamic studies on 11 patients. An injection dose of 0·3 mg/kg was given over 2 min. Immediately after the first minute of injection there was a fall in heart rate and mean blood pressure and at 3 min a decrease in cardiac output. Maximum effects on mean arterial pressure (-27%), cardiac output (-21%), left ventricular work (-52%), and mean pulmonary arterial pressure (-15%) occurred at 15 min. Only the cardiac output returned to the control value at 90 min.

In conclusion, piritramide is useful in intensive care by virtue of its ventilatory depressor effect which facilitate adaptation to the respirator in 81% of cases, which are otherwise difficult to bring under control. Of the 19% who are not adapted, it may be useful for them to have a muscle relaxant such as pancuronium. The symptoms of chronic intoxication in this series of 30 patients were not excessive. These advantages are obtained at the moderate haemodynamic cost of a slight decrease in cardiac output, total systemic resistance and left ventricular work. These results strongly suggest that piritramide may be used safely and profitably in critically ill surgical patients, that prudence is required in case of hypovolemia.

Discussion

T. Savege (London)

If you give the dose every 3 h on average, does that mean that the patient will be with the ventilator for that 3 h period?

P. Glaser

Yes. These patients were on the ventilator for many days.

T. Savege

If they stop breathing against the machine, that is good. But during the 3 h before the next dose, do they make no attempts to breath again?

P. Glaser

We chose a 6 h period so that it was possible to know after 1, 2 or 3 h if they were synchronized with the ventilator. If necessary, the nurse would give another injection. Thus it was possible to know the exact duration of action.

The Effects of Anaesthesia and Surgery on B- and T-Lymphocytes

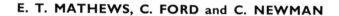

E. T. MATHEWS, C. FORD and C. NEWMAN

Queen Elizabeth Hospital, Birmingham, UK

The phagocytes are stimulated; they devour the disease; and the patient recovers—unless, of course, he's too far gone . . .

George Bernard Shaw

In the preface to his play "The Doctor's Dilemma", George Bernard Shaw was very critical of the medical profession in general, and in particular critical of some of the alleged benefits of anaesthesia. But he did not blame anaesthesia for depressing the phagocytes. Shaw's play was published in 1906 and it was around this period that Rubin (1904) and Graham (1911) described the depressant effect of ether anaesthesia upon the phagocytes. A little later Crile (1913) suggested that ether diminished the immunity of the patient and Gaylord and Simpson (1916) reported that chloroform, and to a lesser extent ether, enhanced the growth of mammary adenocarcinoma in mice.

More recently several investigators using modern anaesthetic agents have shown depression of various parts of the immune defence system and some have compared the degree of depression produced by different agents. One investigation, that of Doenicke and Kropp (1976), found a marked depression in phagocytic activity in a group of patients who had received halothane, nitrous oxide and oxygen, but no depression and even some stimulation of phagocytic activity in a comparable group who were anaesthetized by a technique which they described as neuroleptanalgesia. Whereas previous investigators (Löfström and Schildt, 1974; Cullen *et al.*, 1975) had found differences between groups having these different anaesthetic agents to be small and insignificant. They had used different tests of phagocytic activity. Doenicke had used a lipofundin clearance test; Löfström had used ^{125}I-labelled microaggregates of human serum albumin and their results are in complete conflict. With two of my colleagues, Dr Ford and Dr Newman, I have also studied two groups of patients undergoing surgery and receiving different anaesthetic agents. Using current immunological techniques we have compared the changes in T- and B-lymphocyte counts, changes in the T-lymphocyte subgroup of "active" T-lymphocytes, and changes in the responses to the mitogens phytohaemagglutinin (PHA) and to poke weed mitogen (PWM).

Stress-free Anaesthesia: Royal Society of Medicine International Congress and Symposium Series No. 3, published jointly by Academic Press Inc. (London) Ltd., and the Royal Society of Medicine.

Group A received methohexitone, 75–100 mg, suxamethonium, 50–75 mg or pancuronium 4–8 mg, nitrous oxide, oxygen and halothane 0·5–2·0%.

Group B received methohexitone, 75–100 mg, suxamethonium 50–75 mg or pancuronium 4–8 mg, nitrous oxide, oxygen and fentanyl 0·2–0·4 mg.

Both groups were premedicated with paparvaretum 15 mg and hyoscine 0·3 mg one hour before anaesthesia. The first sample of blood was taken immediately before the induction of anaesthesia and the second sample was taken at the end of surgery and before awakening. All samples were taken between 08·45 and 13·00 hours. The samples were placed in plastic tubes containing preservative free lithium heparin as anticoagulant, and were collected by the immunologist who was not informed of what anaesthetic had been used. The patients chosen for this study were fit and free from conditions such as cardiac disease, cancer, anaemia, or any of the other conditions known to alter the immune responses. All operations were carried out by the same surgical team; there was minimal blood loss, surgery and anaesthesia were uneventful. In no case was blood transfused or dextran given. Burden *et al.*, 1977) have shown that dextran may act as a lymphocyte mitogen. The age groups of the patients and the duration of the procedures were comparable.

There was no significant difference between the pre- and post-anaesthetic counts of total T-cells and B-cells in the two groups. However, there was a statistically significant increase in the number of "active" T-cells in the post-anaesthesia samples of Group A patients, those who had received halothane (Table 1).

Table 1

Capacity of peripheral blood lymphocytes to form T- and B-rosettes

| | % rosette cell formation | | |
	T-cells	"Active" T	B-cells
Group A			
Pre-anaesthesia	70·06	31·35	22·46
Post-anaesthesia	70·10	37·04[a]	21·54
Group B			
Pre-anaesthesia	73·75	33·20	20·52
Post-anaesthesia	73·62	30·75	16·75

[a] $P < 0.05$

As to the ability of lymphocytes to respond to the mitogens PHA and PWM there was a statistically significant difference between the responses in the two groups. There was a reduction in the ability to respond to the mitogen PHA after halothane anaesthesia and this can be taken as evidence of depressed immunological competence (Table 2).

The significance of the increase in the "active" T-cells after halothane is much more difficult to interpret. The "active" T-cells were described by Fudenberg *et al.* (1975) as a subpopulation of T-lymphocytes more actively engaged in cellular immunity than is the total T-cell population. For instance, in some genetically determined immune deficient states the total T-cell population count may be normal but the "active" T-cell population may be low. And when attempts are made to stimulate the immune defences, as with the injection of BCG vaccine into a cutaneous lesion of a patient with malignant melanoma, there can be an increase in the "active" T-cells, again without an effect on the total T-cell count. When levamisole is given to patients they have been shown to display an increase in the level of "active"

Table 2

*Ability of peripheral blood lymphocytes to respond to the
mitogens PHA and PWM*

	Mitogen	
	PHA	PWM
Group A		
Pre-anaesthesia	15,135	2,865
Post-anaesthesia	12,319[a]	2,933
Group B		
Pre-anaesthesia	17,996	3,680
Post-anaesthesia	16,473	3,943

[a]$P < 0.05$

T-cells without an increase in the total T-cell count (Rosenthal, 1977). Thus it appears that the "active" T-cells play an important role in cellular defence.

I have been unable to find any previous work reporting the effects of anaesthesia on the "active" T-cell population, but the stimulation of phagocytes by low dose chloroform was reported as long ago as 1916 (Hamburger). Perhaps this represents another similarity between halothane and chloroform.

In group B, the patients receiving fentanyl, we were unable to show any significant evidence of immunosuppression following anaesthesia and surgery. But the doses of fentanyl used were very small compared with what has been described at this symposium. The dose was 0·4 mg given to fit patients. It is not clear whether a larger dose of fentanyl would have been beneficial. European fentanyl contains ten times the quantity of antifungal drugs, hydroxybenzoates, as preservatives, as it does the active ingredient. Several antifungal drugs have been shown to suppress immune reactivity (Thong, 1977a,b). North American fentanyl is free from this problem and we do not know what the effects of large doses of these preservatives given intravenously would be. The possibility therefore exists that they might have produced immunosuppression had we gone on to use larger drug doses.

The importance of the role of secondary agents in immunological studies is illustrated by a recent report of the depression of the macrophages in mice when the level of chlorine in their drinking water was increased, following an outbreak of infection in the laboratory. Their macrophages could no longer be rendered tumourcidal by macrophage activating factor (Fidler, 1977). When returned to drinking less chlorinated water, the stimulation was again possible.

In 1911, Graham found a simple way to reverse the depression of phagocytes caused by ether; he gave rectal olive oil to his patients and the activity of their phagocytes was restored. As a control he gave others saline per rectum but the depression of their phagocytes continued for several days. Yet by the simple expedient of a little olive oil, phagocytosis was restored. Modern immunology provides more sophisticated methods than this; we have many tests to assess immunologically the effects of anaesthesia and surgery. But it is still very difficult to assess separately the effects of the trauma of the surgeon.

... chloroform has done a lot of mischief. It's enabled every fool to be a surgeon.

George Bernard Shaw

References

Burden, A. C., Stacey, R. L. and Windle, E. *et al.* (1977). *Lancet* **ii**, 688.
Crile, G. W. (1913). *Lancet* **ii**, 7.

Cullen, B. F., Hume, R. B. and Chretien, P. B. (1975). *Anaesthesia and Analgesia* **54,** 501.

Doenicke, A. and Kropp, W. (1976). *British Journal of Anaesthesia* **48,** 1191.

Fidler, I. J. (1977). *Nature* **270,** 735.

Fudenberg, H. H., Wybran, J. and Robbins, D. (1975). *New England Journal of Medicine* **292,** 475.

Gaylord, H. R. and Simpson, B. T. (1916). *Journal of Cancer Research* **1,** 379.

Graham, E. A. (1911). *Journal of Infectious Diseases* **8,** 147.

Hamburger, H. J. (1916). *British Medical Journal* **1,** 37.

Löfström, B. and Schildt, B. (1974). *Acta Anaesthesiologica Scanidnavica* **18,** 34.

Rosenthal, M. (1977). *Lancet* **ii,** 665.

Rubin, G. (1904). *Journal of Infectious Diseases* **1,** 425.

Shaw, G. B. (1906). *The Doctor's Dilemma*. Act 1.

Thong, Y. H. and Rowan-Kelly, B. (1977a). *British Medical Journal* **1,** 149.

Thong, Y. H. and Ness, D. (1977b). *Lancet* **ii,** 568.

Immunological Aspects of Anaesthetic Practice

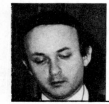

B. WALTON

Anaesthetics Unit, London Hospital, UK

It is becoming increasingly evident that exposure of patients to anaesthesia and surgery adversely affects a whole battery of immune responses. There are a number of factors operating during this period, all of which may have a greater or lesser effect on several facets of immune status. Not only are there both the direct and hormonally-mediated effects of anaesthetic agents themselves, but perhaps more importantly, the hormonal effects of the stress response to anaesthesia and surgery. Other minor factors may also play a part and confuse the picture. For example, coincident therapy such as chloramphenicol and salicylates may have adverse effects on immune responsiveness (Weisberger et al., 1966; Pachmann et al., 1971), blood transfusion alters lymphocyte function (Schechter et al., 1972), and concurrent (perhaps unrecognised) viral infections can depress specific immunity (Notkins et al., 1970). It has even been suggested, although not confirmed, that nutritional deprivation and pyrexia can also have adverse effects.

It has been known since as early as 1896 that patients tend to develop a leucocytosis post-operatively (Von Lerber, 1896). Three years later this leucocytosis was attributed to the anaesthetic agent that was being used at the time, diethyl ether (Chadbourne, 1899). In discussing this problem it is often difficult, if not impossible, to separate the effects of anaesthetic agents on the one hand, from the effects of increased hormone levels on the other, for increases in catecholamines or corticosteroids affect not only the numbers of circulating neutrophils and lymphocytes, but also their efficiency.

It is quite clear that there is interplay between the effects of anaesthetic agents themselves and the influence of alterations in hormone levels in patients during the perioperative period. For example, exposure of animals to diethyl ether will invariably result in leucocytosis. If, on the other hand, they are previously exposed to barbiturates (which prevents the ACTH release usually seen with diethyl ether), the leucocytosis is not seen (Bruce and Wingard, 1971). It has been shown that, in rats, prolonged exposure to nitrous oxide results in leucopenia. However, in wounded or aggressive rats, both of which groups will presumably have high levels of circulating catecholamines and/or steroids, the degree of leucopenia is much more profound (Parbrook, 1967; Green, 1968).

It is clear that hormone levels have tremendously varied effects on several aspects

Stress-free Anaesthesia: Royal Society of Medicine International Congress and Symposium Series N . 3, published jointly by Academic Press Inc. (London) Ltd., and the Royal Society of Medicine.

of immune function. Catecholamines not only increase the numbers of circulating lymphocytes and neutrophils but also alter their distribution and mobilization (Dougherty and Frank, 1953). On the other hand, corticosteroids, although also producing neutrophilia, reduce the number of circulating leucocytes, possibly by a direct toxic effect (Dougherty and Frank, 1953). It has also been shown that, in patients on steroid therapy, phagocytosis is inhibited (Crepea et al., 1951). In addition animal experiments have shown that steroids not only reduce protein synthesis and mitosis but also thymus cell metabolism (Kidson, 1967; Young, 1969). The question to be asked is whether these animal findings are merely of academic interest or whether the levels of hormones seen clinically in the post-operative period would be sufficient to cause these responses.

Exposure to anaesthesia and surgery affects many facets of leucocyte function. Firstly, prolonged exposure to a number of anaesthetic agents, both inhalational and non-inhalational agents, produces a neutropenia. (Lassen et al., 1956; Bruce and Koepke, 1966). This is thought to be related to an inhibition of white cell development in the bone marrow, as it has been shown that both halothane and nitrous oxide delay the maturation of cells in the marrow (Bruce et al., 1971). Secondly, the mobilization of white cells towards the scene of an infection is depressed by a number of anaesthetic agents (Bruce and Wingard, 1971; Bruce, 1967). Thirdly, their motility is reversibly inhibited in a dose-dependent fashion by exposure to halothane (Nunn et al., 1970) and other agents and finally, once they reach the site of infection, their ability to phagocytose foreign particles is inhibited (Bruce, 1967; Graham, 1911).

What are the practical implications of these alterations in immune responses? They relate both to the ability of patients to fight infections in the post-operative period on the one hand and to their ability to come to terms with a pre-existing malignant process on the other.

We will consider infections first. It has been shown that exposure of animals to a number of anaesthetic agents, both inhalational and non-inhalational causes an increase in mortality and morbidity among animals infected with a variety of bacteria (Bruce, 1967; Rubin, 1904; Snel, 1903). The effect of these anaesthetic agents seems to be dose-dependent. Both pulmonary bactericidal activity and the ability of tracheal mucous membranes to expel foreign material are adversely affected by anaesthesia (Goldstein and Munsen, 1971; Lichtiger et al., 1975; Forbes, 1976).

Much less evidence has appeared concerning the effects of exposure to anaesthesia on viral infections, but it seems that anaesthesia may result in increased susceptibility in some species to some viral infections, implying a depressed immune responsiveness. For example, exposure to halothane increases the mortality among mice infected with murine hepatatis virus (Moudgil, 1973).

Perhaps more important, at least from the patients' point of view, is the fact that the delicate balance that may have been established between themselves and their malignant processes may be upset by exposure to anaesthesia and surgery, in a nonspecific way. It is known that immunosuppression favours the spread of malignancy. It is known also that for patients who have had a primary tumour removed some years previously, with no sign of metastatic growth, a coincidental minor surgical procedure such as hernia repair or varicose vein treatment will often cause them to die very quickly from the rapid development of metastases in the post-operative period (Gordon-Taylor, 1948). If tumours are transplanted from one rodent to another, a certain proportion of them will "take". This "take" rate can be increased for transplanted tumours by exposing the hosts not only to a number of anaesthetic agents (Gaylord and Simpson, 1916; Agostino and Cliffton, 1964), but also to varying types of trauma (Buinauskas et al., 1958; Fischer and Fischer, 1959; Gottfried et al., 1961), or indeed, merely by giving them steroids (Gottschalk and Grollman, 1952;

Baserga and Shubik, 1954). A comparison between two groups of women with stage II carcinoma of the breast with respect to annual survival rates, showed that patients who had the relatively non-stressful surgical technique of simple mastectomy survived better than those who had been exposed to the more stressful radical mastectomy (Brinkley and Haybitt, 1966). The degree of stress was apparently relevant in relation to their ability to overcome the threat of metastases, although, of course, many other factors are probably involved.

It is well known that cell-mediated immunity is very important if a patient is to come to terms with malignancy. One of the most commonly used *in vitro* indices of cell-mediated immunity is the lymphocyte transformation test (LTT). It has been shown that the *in vitro* transformation of lymphocytes in response to mitogens is depressed post-operatively (Riddle and Berenbaum, 1967; Park *et al.*, 1971). It is also depressed by exposure to a number of anaesthetic agents (Cullen *et al.*, 1972, Espanol *et al.*, 1974), and by increasing the steroid concentration in the culture medium (McIntyre *et al.*, 1967). Of particular relevance was the report showing that, for three weeks post-operatively, there was a decrease in the patient's ability to mount cell-mediated immune responses against antigens derived from various tumours— irrespective of the anaesthetic agents involved (Cochran *et al.*, 1972).

Although there is a profound decrease in lymphocyte activity *in vitro* in the first few post-operative days, in most patients the level of activity has returned to normal (or even overswung) by the end of the first post-operative week. In patients with malignant disease, however, both the degree of post-operative depression and the duration of that depression may be more marked (Park *et al.*, 1971). It would appear that patients with malignant disease may be particularly at risk from this post-operative immunosuppression.

There is relatively little data comparing one anaesthetic technique with another from the immunosuppressive point of view. Certainly, the data that have appeared and the results from our own Laboratory (which have yet to be published) seem to suggest that there is relatively little to choose between one anaesthetic technique and another. It seems much more likely that the major contributors to post-operative immunosuppression are the hormonal effects of the stress of anaesthesia and surgery, rather than particular anaesthetic agents or techniques themselves. However, certain groups of patients, particularly those with malignant disease, are ill served by being exposed to any form of treatment which unnecessarily depresses their immune responses. In such patients (at least), if it can be shown that totally stress-free anaesthesia minimizes the hormonal changes normally seen during surgery, then such an anaesthetic approach may be of value.

References

Agostino, D. and Cliffton, E. E. (1964). *Archives of Surgery* **88,** 735.
Baserga, R. and Shubik, P. (1954). *Cancer Research* **14,** 12.
Brinkley, D. and Haybitt, J. L. (1966). *Lancet* **2,** 291.
Bruce, D. L. (1967). *Journal of Surgical Research* **7,** 180.
Bruce, D. L. and Koepke, J. A. (1966). *Anesthesiology* **27,** 811.
Bruce, D. L. and Wingard, D. W. (1971). *Anesthesiology* **34,** 271.
Bruce, D. L., Lin, H. S. and Bruce, W. R. (1971). *In:* "Cell Biology and Toxicity of Anesthetics" (Ed. Fink), p 251, Williams and Wilkins, Baltimore.
Buinauskas, P., Macdonald, G. O. and Cole, W. H. (1958). *Annals of Surgery* **148,** 642.
Chadbourne, T. L., (1899). *Philadelphia Medical Journal* **3,** 390.
Cochran, A. J., Spilg, W. C. S., Mackie, R. M. and Thomas, C. E. (1972). *British Medical Journal* **4,** 67.
Crepea, S. B., Magnin, G. E. and Seastone, C. V. (1951). *Proceedings of the Society for Experimental Biology and Medicine* **77,** 704.

78   B. Walton

Cullen, B. F., Sample, W. F. and Chretien, P. B. (1972). *Anesthesiology* **36**, 206.
Dougherty, T. F. and Frank, J. A. (1953). *Journal of Laboratory and Clinical Medicine* **42**, 530.
Espanol, T., Todd, G. B. and Soothill, J. F. (1974). *Clinical Experimental Immunology* **18**, 73.
Fischer, B. and Fischer, E. R. (1959). *Annals of Surgery* **150**, 731.
Forbes, A. R. (1976). *Anesthesiology* **45**, 59.
Gaylord, H. R. and Simpson, B. T. (1916). *Journal of Cancer Research* **1**, 379.
Goldstein, E. and Munson, E. S., cited by Bruce, D. L. and Wingard, D. W. (1971). *Anesthesiology* **34**, 271.
Gordon-Taylor, G. (1948). *Annals of the Royal College of Surgeons* **2**, 60.
Gottfried, B., Molomut, N. and Skaredoff, L. (1961). *Annals of Surgery* **153**, 138.
Gottschalk, R. G. and Grollman, A. (1952). *Cancer Research* **12**, 651.
Graham, E. A. (1911). *Journal of Infectious Diseases* **8**, 147.
Green, C. D. (1968). *Anesthesia and Analgesia: Current Researches* **47**, 509.
Kidson, C. (1967). *Nature (London)* **213**, 779.
Lassen, H. C. A., Henriksen, E., Neukirch, F. *et al.* (1956). *Lancet* **1**, 527.
Lichtiger, M., Landa, J. F. and Hirsch, J. A. (1975). *Anesthesiology* **42**, 753.
McIntyre, O. R., Eurenius, K., Holland, F. C. *et al.* (1967). *Proceedings of Third Annual Leucocyte Culture Conference* (Ed. W. O. Rieke) p.307, Appleton-Century-Crofts, New York.
Moudgil, G. C. (1973). *British Journal of Anaesthesia* **45**, 1236.
Notkins, A. L., Mergehagen, S. E. and Howard, R. J. (1970). *Annals of the Reviews of Microbilology* **24**, 525.
Nunn, J. F., Sharp, J. A. and Kimball, K. L. (1970). *Nature* **226**, 85.
Pachmann, L. M., Easterley, N. B. and Peterson, R. D. A. (1971). *Journal of Clinical Investigation* **50**, 226.
Parbrook, G. D. (1967). *British Journal of Anaesthesia* **39**, 119.
Park, S. K., Brody, J. I., Wallace, H. A. and Blakemore, W. S. (1971). *Lancet* **1**, 53.
Riddle, P. R. and Berenbaum, M. C. (1967). *Lancet* **1**, 746.
Rubin, G. (1904). *Journal of Infectious Diseases* **1**, 425.
Schechter, G. P., Soehnlen, F. and McFarland, W. (1972). *New England Journal of Medicine* **287**, 1169.
Snel, J. J. (1903). *Berlin Klinische Wochenschrift* **40**, 212.
Von Lerber, A. (1896). *Ueber di Einwirkung der Aethernarkose auf Blut und Urin.* Inaugural Dissertation, Bern, Verlags-Druckerei, Basel.
Wesiberger, A. S., Moore, R. D. and Schoenberg, M. D. (1966). *Journal of Laboratory and Clinical Medicine* **67**, 58.
Young, D. A. (1969). *Journal of Biological Chemistry* **244**, 2210.

Discussion

T. Savege (London)

Steroids may depress the stress response but has anyone tried human, post-surgical steroid levels in animal experiments?

B. Walton

No. The doses of steroids used in the experiments mentioned were many times greater than those found clinically, which raises the whole question of whether they are relevant.

But patients on steroid therapy for other reasons do have depressed responses, both specific responses and non-specific resistance mechanisms.

General Discussion

Chairman: R. S. RENEMAN

R. S. Reneman

The main subject of this meeting is *stress-free anaesthesia* and so it is necessary for us to try to define what is meant by *stress*. We have been trying to record phenomena supposedly representative of a situation which itself is not clearly defined. And this is only part of the problem. If we could first agree on what we should try to measure to define a stress-free situation, we then have to resolve the contradictory results reported this morning, which arise presumably from the different combinations of anaesthetics and hypnotics used. This is especially important with regard to immunosuppression, because not only the drug itself, but also the effects of stress, have an important influence on the immunological system.

First then, we should try to define what we mean by stress and to decide whether it is only induced by pain stimuli or also by other stimuli. In other words, even in the presence of adequate analgesia, can stress still exist, for instance because of inadequate hypnosis? Secondly, what do we measure to define stress—metabolic status, catecholamines, blood pressure and heart rate, or all of them?

Thereafter, we have to discuss the action of fentanyl at various doses and say why it is preferable to classical anaesthesia with NLA. An important aspect in this area is the technique of using higher doses, of 8–50 μg/kg. What are the limits of safety, particularly in a general hospital? Looking at Dr Stanley's data, he is clearly justified in his dose regime, if only because his patients will receive assisted ventilation afterwards. But what about the situation which several British workers presented, where they have to discontinue ventilation or where it is not even used? These are some of the areas which I should like to discuss this afternoon.

The Elimination of Stress

C. Prys-Roberts (Bristol)

Could I start by suggesting that we are using the wrong words. We are not talking about *stress-free* but *response-free* anaesthesia, because stress is the perturbation creating the response which we are trying to ablate. Thus, we should avoid the use of the word stress, because we cannot have stress-free anaesthesia unless we do without surgery. The stress is the injury of surgery. It is that injury which produces a series of responses.

Stress-free Anaesthesia: Royal Society of Medicine International Congress and Symposium Series No. 3, published jointly by Academic Press Inc. (London) Ltd., and the Royal Society of Medicine.

They may include the perception of pain and those responses in the defence mechanism for withdrawing from pain. There are also other autonomic hormonal responses to pain and injury which are more long term. When we induce anaesthesia for a surgical operation, we are rendering the patient insensitive to pain.

These other components may occur quite independently, even though the patient may not be aware of them. We have begged the question of whether it is necessary to ablate these responses and this is a question which we really ought to discuss. Many speakers here have shown that by giving high doses of fentanyl or other anaesthetics it is possible to suppress most, if not all, of these responses. But is it necessary in man, or in experimental animals, to ablate a response which is a defence mechanism to injury?

T. Savege (London)

I do not know if it is necessary to suppress these responses, but we must establish whether they matter or not. If we believe that with anaesthesia we are trying to maintain some degree of homeostasis, then we deceive ourselves if we feel that we are achieving that end. Anaesthetists may believe that their patients are not responding to the stimulus of surgery during anaesthesia because they are paralysed, they are pink and they are not sweating. But these are all pharmacological achievements which are not related to the information travelling up and down the central nervous system. Some of us may think that everything is going well, but all of these impulses are actually continuing. It has been said that this is a reflex response protecting the body against assault, but surgery is not a normal physiological assault. I therefore do not fully believe the argument that these responses are absolutely vital for survival.

T. H. Stanley (Salt Lake City)

The administration of a sufficient quantity of almost any opiate will almost totally ablate all the responses to stress that can be measured. The question is therefore whether these ablations are good or not and what are the consequences of high doses of various opiates, other than the ablation of the stress response?

T. Savege

That is correct. There is no doubt that the ablation of the stress response is possible. However, in discussing stress-free anaesthesia we should not only discuss narcotic analgesia. There is work to suggest that one may reduce stress by such techniques as spinal or epidural anaesthesia. It is perhaps more appropriate to alter responses on the afferent limb of the reflex rather than centrally or on the efferent limb. It is only a year or so since we thought the stress response was essential for life. I now believe that in a hospital environment it is not essential, as long as the patient is being looked after by a medical team.

Fentanyl: dosage and side effects

D. Kettler (Goettingen)

Dr Savege believes that an assault on the body occurs in the operating theatre and he is right. But how much fentanyl do you really need to abolish the response? We all want to prevent the patient experiencing pain and a massive responsiveness, with very high blood pressure, for example. But quite moderate doses, for instance 7μg/kg/h, usually prevent a large increase in blood pressure or heart rate during the operation in most cases and do not lead to glucose or lactate production.

T. H. Stanley

In my experience each patient is different and even patients with the same disease process are different among themselves. There is a range and one cannot say that 7 μg/kg/h will be sufficient for every patient, as I am sure you are not. Less will be required by some, greater amounts by others.

T. Savege

I agree with Professor Kettler that one should avoid tachycardias and large rises in blood pressure and I wondered earlier whether *small* changes in cardiovascular dynamics, which might not be harmful for the heart, might give some idea of whether the patient was being stressed. I accept that moderate or small doses of fentanyl would probably provide a stable cardiovascular situation, but they almost certainly will not block hormonal changes. Thus, we come back to the original Chairman's question, *do the hormonal changes matter?* I do not think that we know.

C. Prys-Roberts

It is becoming obvious that fentanyl in man, under conditions of controlled ventilation, has such an enormous therapeutic index that there is no reason why we could not give 100 μg/kg or even 200 μg/kg without producing any harm. The problem comes not in how much we *can* use, but in what it is *appropriate* to use in view of secondary effects, other than analgesia. Most would agree that analgesia *per se* is particularly appropriate as the patient is waking up, but such analgesia is associated with ventilatory depression, irrespective of which opiate drug is used. The patient has inadequate ventilation as a result of using high doses and we can probably get very little further deciding on dosage until one decides what is appropriate management for a particular patient.

When Dr Stanley describes very large doses of fentanyl for heart surgery the doses are entirely appropriate for that type of surgery, for that duration of surgery and because of the fact that he is going to ventilate post-operatively. But for an operation which is going to last 2–3 h, I think it almost essential to reverse some of the effects of the drug at the end of the procedure. I personally would not consider a dose of 50 μg/kg in my elderly patients with vascular disease and 3–4 h operations, because I know that if I use more than 10–15 μg/kg I will have difficulty in establishing post-operative breathing. I would have to reverse the effects by using naloxone and in so doing I would negate part of the benefit already achieved, because it is not easy to reverse the effects of fentanyl by titration.

D. Kettler

I have listed the side effects of high doses of morphine and I would like to establish to what extent they are also seen with fentanyl. The first is respiratory depression, which has been dealt with. The second is antidiuresis.

T. H. Stanley

The addition of nitrous oxide to fentanyl will produce antidiuresis, just as its addition to any anaesthetic technique will produce it. In our comparative study, patients anaesthetized with 2 mg/kg morphine had unchanged cardiovascular dynamics and a vigorous diuresis. Morphine had no effect on urine output or renal function as determined by clearance measurements. With 50% nitrous oxide, however, urine function was reduced by more than 50%. The same happened with fentanyl during anaesthesia, although no-one appears to have studied the phenomenon afterwards

D. Kettler

The third point is muscular rigidity and abnormal muscle movement.

T. H. Stanley

We use a muscle relaxant when the surgical procedure starts, so we do not know if that would be a problem.

D. Kettler

Are there any post-operative psychotic episodes, for example with old patients, using fentanyl in high doses?

T. H. Stanley

Not often. There is no difference between old patients and young patients, in my experience.

K. Peter (*Munich*)

We have the impression that patients with cerebro-vascular disease, often patients 70 years old or more, normally sleep longer with fentanyl. They have psychological problems in the post-operative phase and are not comparable to younger, cerebro-vascular healthy patients, although their $PaCO_2$ is normal.

A. Florence (*Liverpool*)

I have anaesthetized a large number of patients for carotid angiography and carotid endarterectomy, using low doses of fentanyl with droperidol and fentanyl without droperidol. I found that when droperidol had been used with fentanyl they were very disorientated and sometimes completely confused for up to 24 h. But since I stopped using droperidol and used higher doses of fentanyl, I have seen drowsiness but no disorientation.

D. Kettler

Increased blood losses have been reported with increasing morphine doses in cardiopulmonary bypass. Have the same observations been made with high doses of fentanyl?

T. H. Stanley

No. Coronary bypass with 3 h on cardiopulmonary bypass has been achieved with fentanyl in Jehovah's Witnesses whose religion forbids blood transfusion. There is evidence of a venoconstricting effect of fentanyl, in contrast to morphine, which is a venodilating drug.

D. Kettler

At high doses of fentanyl have you ever seen severe hypotension in patients with cardiovascular disease? In a very few of our cases circulation broke down, with bradycardia, a heart rate of less than 60 beats/min in patients who normally display a higher rate.

T. H. Stanley

That is a systemic effect which depends upon the rate of administration and perhaps the volume status of the patient.

T. Savege

This relates to the suppression of stress. Suppressing the stress response will almost certainly stop the body from being able to vasoconstrict in response to a fall in blood volume, since the release of catecholamines and cortisol will be altered. That is probably why patients used to die from not being able to respond to stress in the past. They bled and were not properly transfused. I suspect that a large dose of fentanyl will produce a vaso-dilated patient. If his blood loss is not replaced, he will become very hypotensive. That is obviously a danger of abolishing the stress response.

D. Kettler

Care is required with fluids in some types of patient. One cannot put them into a state of volume overload simply to prevent a fall in blood pressure after a vasodilating agent is injected. It is wise to keep a patient with mitral valve disease, for instance, on somewhat low volume.

T. H. Stanley

I have the impression, looking at the data presented this morning, that the drug has a very transient and minimal effect on peripheral arterial resistance. Nothing was presented about the venous side of the circulation, but from personal experience I suggest that the drug has a minimal effect, if anything venoconstrictor. Thus, theoretically, the only reason that hypotension can occur is because of bradycardia. If bradycardia is avoided, one does not, in my experience, see hypotension.

D. Kettler

It has been reported that under morphine there is a liberation of endo-genous epinephrine and norepinephrine, the so-called *positive inotropic action of morphine*.

C. Conseiller (*Boulogne*)

That was only in the dog, not in man.

D. Kettler

There are two more important comparisons with morphine to be con-sidered. One is a huge increase in bronchomotor tone which can be abolished by a single injection of atropine. The other is the evidence that, in a very few cases, a single high dose of morphine has led to drug dependence.

O. Mayrhofer (*Vienna*)

In our first 50 cases, receiving an average of 50 μg/kg of fentanyl, we were expressly watching for bronchoconstrictor effects but we could not detect any. Occasionally, particularly in children, we saw a rash on the face which might have been a histamine effect, but there was not enough histamine liberated to cause a clinically detectable bronchoconstriction.

C. Prys-Roberts

I do not think that one should be too concerned about these various side effects. They are entirely predictable pharmacological effects shown by all of the drugs which fall into this group. They all produce a vagal action, an acetylcholine-like effect, which will lead to bradycardia and broncho-constriction, to a greater or lesser extent. Rigidity is sometimes observed, more so in other species where lead pipe rigidity is a specific characteristic of opiate drugs. And what may be taken for bronchoconstriction or bronchospasm may simply be a rigidity of the chest wall which will be detected as a decrease in the ability to inflate the lungs,

R. S. Reneman

Recent studies of Dr de Castro and co-investigators on neurovegetative stimulation of morphinomimetics in the dog showed that at low doses, vagal stimulation was predominant. Sympathetic stimulation started at relatively low doses and increased with dosage. For fentanyl there was equilibrium between parasympathetic and sympathetic stimulation at doses between $10\,\mu g/kg$ i.v. and $2\,mg/kg$ i.v. This margin is wide, as compared to that for morphine (30–60 mg/kg i.v.) and phenoperidine (0·3–6 mg/kg i.v.).

Fentanyl: mode of administration

M. Zindler (*Dusseldorf*)

On the question of tolerance, it makes a considerable difference whether the drug is given as a bolus injection or slowly, as an infusion. A bolus injection may have an enormous effect at the receptor site, which may cause difficulties. We have not seen chest wall rigidity, for example, for a long time, probably because of slow administration. In discussing high doses, this should be stressed. If bradycardia does occur, however, it can easily be corrected by atropine and hypotension avoided if action is taken immediately.

T. H. Stanley

I confirm Professor Zindler's observations. After establishing the drug in the blood stream by slow infusion, a tolerance is seen in the bradycardic response so that a bolus dose will not then evoke a bradycardia. The situation is similar in man and in the dog. After a dose of 3 mg/kg in the dog to establish the blood level, the bradycardic response to usual stimulants was completely absent. In man, the initial infusion takes about 5 min, at an infusion rate of 100–300 $\mu g/litre$.

J. Crul (*Nijmegen*)

In Philadelphia I studied two groups of identical orthopaedic patients, one given i.v. doses of fentanyl, the other i.m. doses, 1·5 times as large. None of the i.m. patients had muscular ridigity, but it was seen in a large proportion of those with the i.v. dose. The rate of increase of blood concentration is thus impor tant for the development of muscle rigidity.

R. S. Reneman

In attempting to avoid unwanted side effects, high blood pressure, for example, is it appropriate to administer fentanyl incrementally, or should we use high doses at the outset?

D. Kettler

We have used incremental administration but we now use only infusion analgesia with an infusion machine. We changed out technique because we found that it led to smoother haemodynamics and also permitted the average dose to be decreased. Previously we had to give 0·5 mg i.v. for a healthy individual, repeated every 30 min, up to 0·75 mg. We now need only 65 % of this, using infusion analgesia and we have the same level of analgesia as with the higher incremental doses. I believe that one should use only as much drug as the patient needs whilst remaining free from sweating or heart rate or blood pressure increases.

R. S. Reneman

Why should a reduced infusion dose produce a similar effect to a larger bolus dose and what is the relation between CNS binding and plasma concentration?

W. Soudijn (Amsterdam)

The pharmacokinetics are so difficult that I do not have an answer to the first question. As to the second we know that fentanyl is bound to opiate receptors in the central nervous system and also to other specific regions. By contrast, morphine is not so much bound to these specific CNS areas, only to the opiate receptors. Since fentanyl is also at sites near the opiate receptors there is, of course, a dynamic equilibrium. This might explain its unexpectedly long duration of action, but not the infusion effect.

T. Savege

I have given bolus doses of 20 μg/kg and I had three patients out of about eight who developed a massive tachycardia, with the heart rate rising from 70 to about 150 some 40 min later. I have no explanation for this effect which does not seem to relate to surgical stimulus since it is far larger than the tachycardia normally seen in relation to surgery.

A. Florence

Several times I have seen a tachycardia more than doubling heart rate at about 45 min after either 20 or 25 μg/kg of fentanyl, though not at lower doses. I gave an increment of fentanyl, without much success. The condition subsequently subsided.

T. Savege

With my old techniques of analgesia I gave increments far more often. Now I am not giving them for 45–50 min intervals and I wonder whether the patient could be waking up. To reduce the tachycardia I have been giving small doses of intravenous agents but I do not know whether the two facts are related.

K. Peter

Is there any evidence of fentanyl ion channels being responsible for the effects which depend upon rate of administration?

W. Soudijn

The question is difficult. On starting an infusion, the body does not know that this is to be an infusion or how many channels are open.

D. Kettler

A bolus injection of the drug will decline exponentially and there will be a level where analgesia is needed again. The practical working anaesthetist, if he does not see the patient sweating or experiencing an increased heart rate, will repeat the dose every 30 min because this is standard procedure, irrespective of whether anaesthesia is light or deep at that moment. But an infusion, delivering at a constant rate, may keep the patient just above a certain threshold level. It may thus not only be a question of pharmacokinetics but of the practical behaviour of the anaesthetist.

W. Soudijn

But a bolus dose should overshoot the capacity of the liver to metabolize it and leave more drug available to act. The measurement of plasma levels might help to provide the solution.

M. Zindler

Metabolism per unit time is dependent on the total dose. With a high dose, more is metabolized than with a low dose. Thus, with continuous infusion, less drug may be broken down per unit time.

W. Soudijn

This will depend upon the amount of enzyme present.

D. Duvaldestin (*Paris*)

If the clearance of the drug is limited by active transport or by biotransformation, then an increase in plasma concentration during continuous infusion will occur when the dose exceeds the ability of the liver to specific biotransformation and/or biliary excretion of this drug. In contrast, if the drug is eliminated without active transport, there will be no accumulation, and excretion will run parallel to plasma concentration and dosage. For a drug that is metabolized, there is theoretically an upper limit to drug metabolism corresponding to the Vmax of the enzyme responsible for the biotransformation which is concerned. If the concentration achieved during continuous infusion exceeds the Vmax condition, then accumulation will occur. If the hepatic metabolism or biliary elimination of the drug is not saturable, one would expect no accumulation during continuous infusion.

R. S. Reneman

It is a frequent observation that the effects of chronic administration of drugs may be relateable to plasma levels, but acute administration far less often.

T. H. Stanley

With opiate techniques, especially in patients who have a propensity to hypertension, most workers have observed hypertension and tachycardia, especially after open heart surgery. We rarely see it with either morphine or fentanyl because our rate of administration gives more of a bolus effect than a slow constant infusion. The patient receives a higher level of drug than that which will allow breakthrough. Once haemodynamic breakthrough occurs its reversal is very difficult. This is one of the dangers of trying to give *just enough* fentanyl or morphine.

Given a drug with a large therapeutic safety index, it is better to use a larger quantity at the outset. It may be an erroneous concept to want to give just enough. It seems preferable to give more than enough to avoid subsequent complications. In the doses that I am using, it is no longer a short acting drug. But, in my opinion, the only detrimental effect is respiratory depression (less, incidentally, than that seen with morphine) which one should be equipped to handle and which is therefore of no concern.

J. Crul

The vagal stimulation caused by fentanyl occasionally resets the whole balance of sympathetic and parasympathetic tone. At a given moment there may be an overshoot of sympathetic stimulation producing tachycardia. By keeping above a low level there is no breakthrough, but one can not ignore the post-operative complications seen on higher doses.

T. H. Stanley

Post-operatively, the only complication is the need to respirate these patients, who would probably have to be respirated even on lower doses. In addition, there is too much individual patient variability to say arbitrarily that a particular dose will be adequate. Since I do not have enough experience to say exactly what the individual's response will be, I err on the side of avoiding a sympathetic breakthrough. At this moment, I have no alternative.

Fentanyl: mode of Action and interactions

R. Dudziak (Frankfurt)

During neuroleptanalgesia, we cannot generally conclude that there exists a direct relationship between catecholamine levels in plasma and the degree of analgesia or pain. In 80 patients with cardiopulmonary bypass we have investigated the level of plasma catecholamines, temperature and $PaCO_2$ after injection of 0·5 mg of fentanyl. At a temperature of 36°C and a blood $PaCO_2$ of 38 torr we found adrenaline levels of 135 ng/litre and noradrenaline of 198 ng/litre during neuroleptanalgesia. Simply lowering the temperature whilst maintaining the same level of analgesia produced sympathetic activity. For example, at 33°C we found an increase in adrenaline from 135 to 665 ng/litre and in noradrenaline from 289 to 726 ng/litre with an increase in peripheral resistance. At this temperature of 33°C, we also altered the $PaCO_2$ to 17 torr. We found that if the $PaCO_2$ was high, adrenaline and noradrenaline levels and the activity of dopamine beta-hydroxylase were also high. Thus, during surgery under fentanyl analgesia, several situations independent of the state of analgesia will stimulate catecholamine production. They include a fall in temperature, changes in $PaCO_2$ and drug interaction.

T. Savege

That is correct. Included within the so called stress response are a number of physiological changes such as hypothermia, hypoxia, hypotension and noxious stimulation. I believe that the stress response is an adverse response and that if one sees a patient with changing heart rate or blood pressure one should search for the stressing agent which may be the impact of surgery, or some other factor. Normally, of course, anaesthetists have these other factors under control. They measure body temperature and they have the capacity to measure $PaCO_2$ and to transfuse blood. In routine surgery, with these other factors controlled the catecholamine change will normally be due to the noxious stimulus.

R. Dudziak

We have demonstrated that changes in catecholamine level are very sensitive to changes in blood gases. A change in $PaCO_2$ between 30 and 40 torr produces a change in catecholamine level of 300 ng/litre. If other factors are held constant, fentanyl administration *per se* does not influence catecholamine levels, but with surgical stress, the levels increase. It is interesting to note that the action of fentanyl on the pain after this surgical stress is reduced, due perhaps to an interaction between fentanyl and adrenaline receptors. The doses were 2–3 mg per patient before bypass and 0·5 mg per patient during the bypass period.

T. H. Stanley

In this situation fentanyl is being used as a supplement rather than the primary agent, which leads to a different set of effects.

T. Savege

Although the patients on bypass are given droperidol, the possibility exists that by keeping CO_2 low they are being kept unconscious but allowing CO_2 to increase towards normal may cause the patients to wake up.

R. S. Reneman

In trying to avoid unwanted side effects we have so far discussed blood pressure, heart rate, blood gases and temperature, which can be measured continuously. But how can we be sure that if these are constant then glucose metabolism, for example, or the immunological system are also functioning normally?

T. H. Stanley

We have measured only a few other parameters. One is antidiuretic hormone which, in our hands, is very well correlated with the change in dynamics. To avoid the stresses of surgery by using morphine, the dosage has to be very high and the complications of, for example, severe respiratory depression are real. With fentanyl, such complications are less apparent.

T. Savege

We are undertaking a study which attempts to correlate variation in heart rate against hormonal changes. It is difficult because the time response of various measurements is quite different. Catecholamine and sympathetic nervous system activity is almost instantaneous, but ACTH and cortisol take about 30 min to rise after a stressing signal, the duration and intensity of which is itself not fully established. Despite the difficulties, there is no doubt that with 20 μlitres/kg of fentanyl, cortisol, ACTH and growth hormone levels are raised at 40 min although we do not have data on what happens before that.

R. S. Reneman

I would also put a question to Dr Hall and Dr Florence who reported contradictory results. Was this due to different doses of fentanyl, or to combination with different hypnotics?

A. Florence (*Liverpool*)

Despite the fact that we are trying to avoid the term, it may be due to different degrees of surgical stress.

G. Hall (*London*)

We should recognize that we have investigated one model only. Attempts to transpose particular results from mitral stenotic patients to vascular patients or gynaecological patients are obviously not valid. All that I may conclude is that in my particular patients having a particular operation, 50 μg/kg of fentanyl ablates the cortisol, growth hormone and hyperglycaemic responses. But this may not apply to arterial or cardiac surgery.

Different problems exist, in those spheres, in relation to fluid balance, for example. Several authors showed blood losses of up to 4 litres and Dr Dudziak has shown that changes in temperature and CO_2 effect plasma catecholamine levels. Unless one can devise a comparable study with these factors controlled or in some way compensate for them, strict comparisons are impossible. Even worse, cortisol response has a 45 min latent period and growth hormone appears to be similar. Thus, I suspect that even trying to correlate hormonal with cardiovascular changes will itself be extremely difficult.

C. Prys-Roberts

One most important issue, which has to be discussed when talking about side effects, is the question of post-anaesthetic ventilatory depression. If we give doses as large as Dr Stanley then we may expect either to have to reverse them with naloxone or to have to ventilate the patient. Many patients given high doses of fentanyl will breathe spontaneously either with a CO_2 challenge or perhaps with reversal by an antagonist, but a small proportion do develop serious ventilatory depression some time after intensive care has been withdrawn, i.e. after they have left the recovery room. A recent report from Oxford (Adams and Pybus, 1978) described three patients given modest doses of fentanyl who recovered perfectly well, but suddenly stopped breathing on going back to the ward. The problem was recognized. They were treated with naloxone and they recovered.

But there is a serious question here. Depending on the doses used during anaesthesia, we should be able to predict from the pharmacokinetics, particularly the blood levels, the outcome after a particular time in a reasonably large cross-section of the population. I therefore wonder if the blood level of fentanyl is the variable that we should be measuring as a means of detecting adverse effects. Ventilatory depression implies a binding of fentanyl to the neurones in the medulla. That binding must be very rapid because as soon as a bolus dose of fentanyl is given, ventilatory depression may occur. Professor Soudijn informs me that the cerebrospinal fluid level of fentanyl does not rapidly follow the blood level. There may be a phase lag of up to 60 min. Thus it is conceivable that if there are high levels in the CSF (and Professor Soudijn was describing levels of 4 ng/ml), then the CSF pool of fentanyl could act as a potential source of ventilatory depression, as opposed to the vascular pool.

W. Soudijn (*Amsterdam*)

In four patients given 30 μg/kg of fentanyl, the maximum plasma level was 300 ng/ml. The CSF level in two patients almost reached 4 ng/ml at 10–40 min after the peak serum level was achieved. The other two patients had peak levels of 1·5 ng/ml. It is therefore possible that ventilatory depression might be caused by an extremely high CSF level and perhaps by measuring CSF levels (at least as a research investigation) directly after the operation, we might be able to predict side effects.

J. Crul

There is another possibility for the late respiratory depressant effects of these drugs. There may be inactive receptor sites in the body which have a large enough volume to store some of the fentanyl and release it later. This has been shown for muscle relaxants, particularly in cartilage and in bone.

With the newer steroid relaxants we showed a similar storing effect in the liver. Up to 60% of the total dose after 30 min was accumulated in the liver, then later liberated into the blood stream. Total body radiography studies of fentanyl might show inactive receptor sites in which there is no real breakdown of the product, but which could free the fentanyl after a few hours.

R. S. Reneman

What drugs did the four patients with high CSF levels of fentanyl receive in addition to fentanyl itself?

W. Soudijn

They were given diazepam 5 mg and atropine sulphate 0·4 mg for pre-medication. Anaesthesia was induced with i.v. sodium pentothal 3–4 mg/kg and maintained with nitrous oxide, 60–70% inspired air concentration. Pancuronium 0·1 mg/kg was injected prior to tracheal intubation and respiration was controlled with a mechanical ventilator. Thereafter, they received the doses of fentanyl.

C. Prys-Roberts

One other possibility for post-anaesthetic ventilatory depression, in those patients who would almost inevitably have been artificially ventilated during anaesthesia and surgery, depends on whether the PCO_2 had fallen to a low level, as a result of which there had been a substantial loss of CO_2 stores from the body. There have been a number of studies of CO_2 responsiveness in patients who have been given varying doses of fentanyl with or without droperidol. Investigators in San Francisco (Harper *et al.*, 1976) showed that a dose of 9 μg/kg of fentanyl would produce a depression of the CO_2 response curve down to about 40% of normal just before awakening, but with a complete reversal to normality very shortly after-wards. However, at about 40–60 min post-operatively, the CO_2 response curve again appeared to be considerably flattened, down to about 50% of the control value. Unfortunately, in that particular study, none of the patients had a $PaCO_2$ higher than 40 and even though the CO_2 response curve was flattened some time after the termination of anaesthesia, so there was no evidence that it was associated with ventilatory depression. The patients were ventilated with a normal $PaCO_2$ throughout.

I would suggest that if patients have been over-ventilated and the CO_2 has been washed out, according to studies by Sullivan (Sullivan *et al.*, 1966) in New York which showed that it takes 1–2 h for the body CO_2 stores to come back to normal, the decreased CO_2 body store may coincide with a time when the CO_2 response curve is flat. This might be the time when a depressed CO_2 response curve would be associated with ventilatory depression and consequent hypoxia.

R. Cookson (*Marlow*)

I agree. Obviously the CO_2 levels are very important and if investigators are going to make these types of study I would like to make a plea that they try to keep them as simple as possible. Several of the studies presented today, particularly from the UK, involve the use of long-acting opiates as premedication. Whatever their benefits, one result is that they largely invalidate any study of fentanyl itself. Any additional drug could have effects, for example, on $PaCO_2$ levels. The three patients in Oxford who had respiratory depression appearing some time after surgery had opiate premedication, two with papaveritum and one with morphine.

P. Glaser

Sullivan's findings related to hypoxaemia only 60 min after operation.

C. Prys-Roberts

That is true but I am suggesting that this could coincide with a time in these patients when the CO_2 response curve was depressed. Sullivan's patients were not subject to ventilatory depression by other drugs. Theirs was simply a secondary effect of CO_2 washout and the fact that it takes a long time to build up adequate CO_2 body stores. In patients who have had high doses of fentanyl that 60 min might be extended considerably and this may be the danger.

M. Zindler

It is very important to stress the potential dangers of high doses of fentanyl, especially in short cases or in institutions which do not employ routine ventilation after operations. The use of large doses might cause problems because of unpredictable factors such as differences in blood level. At Dr Stanley's doses I also think it is dangerous to use an antidote. Immediately after giving it, the patient is awake and oriented, but 20 min later when the naloxone no longer acts he may become unconscious and if he is not closely observed he may have severe respiratory depression. We should state very clearly that such treatment with high doses of fentanyl can only be performed with certain precautions and that a number of features have to be watched very closely.

T. H. Stanley

In addition, this technique is not meant for every patient. Fentanyl in large doses is perhaps the preferred technique for patients with cardiovascular instability. For patients without this problem, there are many other good anaesthetic techniques that do not occasion the need to ventilate for long periods of time. I assume that I am going to ventilate my patients because post-operative ventilation is desirable for them. But if the patient has a healthy myocardium there are many other techniques available, both intravenous and inhalation, which may be just as good if not better, especially if facilities for post-operative mechanical ventilation and assessment of respiratory status are not readily available.

T. Savege

We do not know whether stress is good or bad, but it is very likely that for a healthy man any harmful effects of the stress response may not matter. The dangers of trying to obliterate the stress response with very large doses of narcotics might therefore outweigh the advantages. Perhaps only in patients who are severely traumatized and undergoing a long period of intensive care will stress suppression make sense, starting at the time of surgery and going through the intensive care period.

R. S. Reneman

On Dr Stanley's point about cardiovascular activity, we have recently completed a study on the effect of fentanyl on myocardial metabolism and left ventricular haemodynamics in dogs with 70–75% coronary artery stenosis. During ischaemia pretreatment with fentanyl, 25 $\mu g/kg$ i.v., resulted in a reduction by 50% in lactate production, as compared to ischaemia without fentanyl, for a similar glucose-uptake. The study indicates that fentanyl decreases anaerobic glycolis possibly due to a decreased oxygen demand. The fall in local pH due to the coronary artery

stenosis was significantly less pronounced when the animals were pre-
treated with fentanyl and this reduction in hydrogen ion concentration in
the ischaemic myocardium will be beneficial for cardiac muscle performance.

D. Kettler

Dogs need. large doses of fentanyl otherwise one can not anaesthetize
them. Man does not need such high doses. Even so, we have found that
the survival time after controlled hypoxia is much higher for dogs with
fentanyl anaesthesia than with halothane. All animals died rapidly from
rhythm disorders and circulatory breakdown after halothane. Survival
time was, however, about 21 min with fentanyl, piritramide or any other
opiate anaesthetic. If a beta-blocking agent is added before the hypoxia,
survival can be prolonged to 63 min. Tolerance to hypoxia and ischaemia
are therefore much better with this type of anaesthesia than with anything
we have had before.

R. S. Reneman

Ischaemia is even more dangerous than hypoxia, because in hypoxia it is
possible to wash out metabolic products locally from the myocardium.

M. Zindler

Is this a specific cardiac effect or is it a more general effect on metabolism,
perhaps an oxygen-sparing phenomenon?

D. Kettler

It is certainly not a question of reducing overall body metabolism, because
it is very difficult to lower metabolism below a certain level with any kind
of anaesthesia. In dogs, one cannot fall below 4 ml/kg/min of oxygen,
whatever additional doses of inhalational or other anaesthetics are used.
But cardiovascular stability is much greater with neuroleptanaesthesia
than with other methods. Negative inotropism is much less pronounced,
even in the ischaemic heart.

R. S. Reneman

I wish to return to Dr Cookson's point about the combination of other
drugs with fentanyl, especially morphinomimetics, muscle relaxants and
hypnotics. Is it likely that some of the post-operative ventilation problems
(which are not very common) are due to premedication with other opiates?

A. Florence

I do not premedicate my patients at all and have still seen $PaCO_2$ values
between 56 and 75 for the post-operative period, although not in combination with droperidol. Two of the three respiratory arrests had periods
of apnoea or very depressed respiration, following the inadvertent administration of an unnecessary dose of analgesic by the nursing staff who
felt the patient should receive it because his pulse rate and blood pressure
had been stable for 30 min.

C. Prys-Roberts

In discussing interactions with other agents it is worth mentioning a
technique which we use fairly widely. A modest dose of fentanyl, 12–15
μg/kg, is combined with a slow infusion of the steroid anaesthetic Althesin.
Both fentanyl and Althesin are profound ventilatory depressants but their

effects are not simply additive. The depressant effect of fentanyl is predominantly on rate. A patient with a high blood concentration of fentanyl will take deep breaths at a slow rate. However, in common with the inhalational agents, Althesin will depress minute volume, but if anything will increase rate. The combined effect of Althesin and fentanyl is to decrease both rate and tidal volume. Normally we use these drugs with controlled ventilation throughout anaesthesia. Althesin is so short-lasting that we can detect no residual overlay of ventilatory depression beyond that which we would expect from fentanyl alone. But anyone using the two drugs with spontaneous breathing must remember that they act in this additive way.

D. Kettler

When using a hypnotic like Althesin or etomidate, is it still necessary to have a high dose of fentanyl or will the addition of a hypnotic produce the same response at a lower dose because of some interaction?

C. Prys-Roberts

When using Althesin with the added analgesia of fentanyl, very high doses of fentanyl are not necessary. The reason that Dr Stanley does not use Althesin is that he cannot obtain it in America. But, apart from etomidate and Althesin, there are no other substances which can be used for continuous infusion without any degree of accumulation and without circulatory depression.

T. H. Stanley

The drugs that we have used in combination with fentanyl are limited but diazepam and nitrous oxide change the picture. However, I would like to know whether cardiac output is unchanged when mixing fentanyl with etomidate or Althesin.

C. Prys-Roberts

We have not studied that question with etomidate. But with althesin there is a minimal degree of reduction in blood pressure and cardiac output on adding a high or moderate dose of fentanyl to a continuing infusion of althesin and vice versa.

R. S. Reneman

No interference was found between fentanyl and etomidate, at least as far as systolic and diastolic aortic pressure and some respiratory functions are concerned. Fentanyl, however, potentiates the increase in heart rate and the decrease in pH after etomidate as well as the duration of sleep induced by this hypnotic.

T. Savege

Althesin augments fentanyl only in so far as Althesin provides unconsciousness. One is eliminating a source of stress through the cortex in making the patient unconscious, when presumably to produce unconsciousness with fentanyl would require a very large dose. But I do not believe that Althesin suppresses stress in any way. To suppress stress responses arising from physiological and pathological changes in the body, one requires a large dose of fentanyl as well as Althesin.

R. S. Reneman

Do the majority of those present favour the use of an hypnotic in combination with fentanyl, or do they prefer to give very high doses of fentanyl itself? Most of the speakers seemed to express a preference for a hypnotic.

T. Savege

I like the idea which Professor Crul mentioned of balanced anaesthesia, where one titrates the three different modalities of stopping responses to noxious stimulation, providing sleep and providing muscle relaxation. I believe that one should provide just enough sleep to keep the patient unconscious, enough muscle relaxant to make surgery possible and convenient and enough analgesia to prevent noxious responses. But how much drug is required to stop them, we still do not know.

M. Zindler

Dr Stanley, why did you use diazepam?

T. H. Stanley

We used it in the early part of our study because we were not sure that we could achieve amnesia even with very high doses of fentanyl. Subsequently we stopped using it and no patient of the 50–100 in the series has ever had inadequate amnesia. My own personal experience would suggest that a hypnotic is unnecessary. In my opinion, I am also blocking all parameters of the stress response, without confusing the issue. Respiratory depression is minimal since patients will be mechanically ventilated for approximately 2–3 h, and we assume that we will ventilate every patient who receives the technique.

T. Savege

None of us actually knows, in our so-called paralyzed patients, whether they are awake or asleep. Many publications in the literature on nitrous oxide relaxant anaesthesia show that the patient had been aware during the procedure. Although he may have subsequently forgotten it, the experience can nonetheless modify the whole of his future life. I am therefore developing the idea of providing hypnosis with i.v. althesin and using the cerebral function monitor which has clear landmarks with i.v. hypnotics but does not have clear landmarks with fentanyl or nitrous oxide.

M. Zindler

The general feeling of those here who have experience with large doses of fentanyl is that with these doses the patient will not recall anything during the induction, particularly the intubation. In this it differs from high doses of morphine. Some of our morphine patients had recollections and had very disagreeable hallucinations when they were half awake. We have not seen this with high doses of fentanyl.

T. H. Stanley

It is simply a matter of dosage. With morphine at 2–3 mg/kg some patients will remember. At 7–9 mg/kg none will do so. However, the complications are too great to tolerate that dosage. With 70–100 μg/kg of fentanyl, however, we have the equivalent of 7–8 mg/kg of morphine without side effects.

M. Kettler

I would like to ask one final question. How does one know that 50 μg/kg, not 10 or 25 or 100 μg/kg, is optimum?

T. H. Stanley

The lowest dose that I have used is about 60–65 μg/kg for total procedure; 50 is my starting level. We have pursued this question in every possible way at our disposal, asking the patients, for example, *are you sure you did not feel anything: are you sure you do not remember any particular sounds?* Thus, I know that the dosages that we have used are adequate. By erring on the high side I cover all eventualities. As to 100 μg/kg, that is the dose that we started with.

O. Mayrhofer

I believe, with Professor Kettler, that we should not overload our patients with very high doses of any single drug. My colleagues in cardiac anaesthesia in Vienna, who five years ago used 50 μg/kg of fentanyl, have returned to the use of a small induction dose of droperidol with no hypnotic. They hardly ever use more than 20 μg/kg body weight now. Indeed, they are already reducing the dose of fentanyl again. They do, however, also use nitrous oxide.

J. Crul

We should warn those who read this discussion not to use this technique for the ordinary patient. It should be reserved for special occasions or special operations because of the dramatic influence it could have on the organization of our post-operative care. If we had to ventilate 70% of our post-operative patients, this could cause a dramatic breakdown of post-operative care, both in the recovery room and in the intensive care unit.

R. S. Reneman

That will be true for doses of 50 μg/kg, but it is also likely to occur at lower doses.

References

Adams, A. P. and Pybus, D. A. (1978). *British Medical Journal* **1**, 278.
Harper *et al.* (1976). *Journal of Pharmacology and Experimental Therapeutics* **199**, 464.
Sullivan, S. F., Patterson, R. W. and Papper, E. M. (1966). *Journal of Applied Physiology* **21**, 247.

Chairman's Summing up

R. S. RENEMAN

Department of Physiology, University of Limburg,
Maastricht, Netherlands

I shall now attempt the difficult task of summarizing the contributions.

First, whether we ourselves are using high doses (in the order of 50 μg/kg) or doses of 10–20 μg/kg (which the average anaesthetist is now working with) we know that it is safe to give high doses during the period of the operation. Post-operative problems can occur with high dose administration and we are not sure at which dose the problem starts. This question will have to be investigated further. Fortunately, it is only a relatively small proportion of patients who suffer respiratory depression post-operatively, but they have to be watched for even this involves some reorganisation of the intensive care facilities.

Secondly, the side effects of even high doses of fentanyl can be predicted and treated directly. One of the advantages of fentanyl over morphine is that histamine release only occurs at very high fentanyl doses, which is not the case with morphine. Certainly, from the possible side effects listed by Dr Kettler and discussed by Dr Stanley and others, fentanyl side effects are few during the operation period.

During the operation we all agree on the need to keep blood pressure, heart rate, temperature and blood gases as stable as possible. It has been shown that fentanyl suppresses the responses to stress. Although it is likely that the dose required depends on the degree of stimulation of the autonomic nervous system, we do not yet know which dose will prevent the breakthrough in blood pressure, heart rate and other variables. Nor do we understand the correlation between the stability of these variables and, for example, metabolic changes or immunological systems. We must decide whether such changes are really important.

Certainly lactate, pyruvate, cortisol and ACTH remained stable in some studies during fentanyl anaesthesia. But would a small increase in lactate, for example, be deleterious, since the ischaemic heart might benefit from it? The consensus view of anaesthetists here is to combine fentanyl with a hypnotic, unless one can prove that very high doses of fentanyl actually produce hypnosis and amnesia. If so, it might strengthen the case for using the doses suggested by Dr Stanley for open heart surgery, where post-operative ventilation is anticipated. The necessity of combining fentanyl with adequate doses of muscle relaxants is agreed upon.

Various hypotheses have been formulated to explain the recurrent post-operative

Stress-free Anaesthesia: Royal Society of Medicine International Congress and Symposium Series No. 3 published jointly by Academic Press Inc. (London) Ltd.. and the Royal Society of Medicine.

respiratory depressant effects of fentanyl. First, there is a possible relationship with the high levels of fentanyl in the CSF. Secondly, there may be a delayed redistribution of fentanyl from the central or peripheral stores. Finally, there may be a decreased responsiveness to CO_2 after the operation.

If we wish to pursue these problems, then we should not forget, for example, that morphinomimetics have a protective effect on the ischaemic myocardium in hypoxia. We would like to have your suggestions on the direction of future studies on fentanyl, to produce an agreed protocol for joint collaboration.

I should like to thank all contributors for their papers, and for their contributions to the discussions. I do not believe that we have ignored any important aspects of the subject. And a final thanks should be said to the Janssen Research Foundation.